The
TRUTH
ABOUT
Breast
CANCER

A ⑦-STEP
PREVENTION PLAN

JOSEPH KEON Ph.D.
RECIPES BY JEAN-MARC FULLSACK

PARISSOUND PUBLISHING

NOTICE TO THE READER

The information presented in this book is by no means intended to replace the advice of your personal physician. The author does not directly or indirectly dispense medical advice or prescribe the use of diet as a means of treating disease without prior medical approval. If you are seriously ill, please do not make any dietary changes or begin any type of exercise program without first consulting your medical doctor. The author and publisher make no claims as to being able to prevent, treat, or cure any form of cancer or other disease and assume no responsibility for the health of the reader.

Parissound Publishing
16 Miller Avenue
Mill Valley, CA 94941
(888) 544-LIFE

Publisher's Cataloguing-in-Publication
(Provided by Quality Books, Inc.)
Keon, Joseph.
    The truth about breast cancer: a seven-step prevention plan/Joseph Keon.–1st ed.
        p. cm.
    Includes bibliographical references and index
    Preassigned LCCN: 94-12045
    ISBN: 0-9648974-7-4

    1. Breast—Cancer—Prevention. 2. Breast—Cancer—Epidemiology. I. Title.

RC280.B8K46 1998   616.99'449'052
                                    QBI98-933

Cover design: Dunn & Associates
Typography: Paula Doubleday Design
Illustrations: Jim Balkovek

Manufactured in the United States of America.
10 9 8 7 6 5 4 3 2 1

OCT 9 '99

This book is dedicated to women the world over, whose lives it may help to save, and to the millions of women for whom this information came too late.

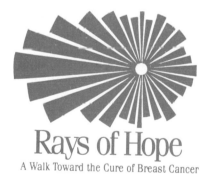

Rays of Hope
A Walk Toward the Cure of Breast Cancer

"The Truth About Breast Cancer is an eye-opening examination of a feared health menace—and a potent action plan for reducing cancer risk while improving health in every respect."

—Michael Klaper, M.D.
   Institute for Nutrition Education and Research
   Author of *Vegan Nutrition: Pure and Simple*

"The Truth About Breast Cancer is a practical guide for all women wishing to reduce their future risk of this dreaded disease. The writing is definitive, well researched, and understandable. The recipes will be invaluable for those seeking better health through delicious food."

—John McDougall, M.D.
   Author of *The McDougall Plan* and
   McDougall's Medicine: A Challenging Second Opinion

"The Truth About Breast Cancer is outstanding! This is a book that clearly, carefully, and accurately shows you how to dramatically reduce your risk of cancer. But that's not all. Heeding its council will bring countless other benefits. Your body will thank you for the rest of your life."

—John Robbins
   Author of *Reclaiming Our Health* and
   Diet For a New America

"The Truth About Breast Cancer is a comprehensive guide for all women of all ages—well researched and referenced, and a great contribution to society."

—Helen Caldicott, M.D.
   Co-founder of Physicians for Social Responsibility
   Author of *If You Love This Planet*

"I strongly recommend that you look at this book if you want to truly educate yourself or someone else about this threatening disease in a way that gets beyond the mainstream aphorisms and into the real causes of and ways to prevent breast cancer."

—Patricia Dines
Community Action Publications

Contents

Foreword

Imagine waking up to read the morning newspaper and discovering that while you slept, a commercial jet had crashed killing all 130 passengers aboard. The newspaper headline might report, *"Tragedy Strikes."* Reading further, you would be assured to know that the National Transportation Safety Board (NTSB) was already on the scene attempting to determine the cause of this fatal disaster.

Indeed, when such an event occurs, nothing can be done for the victims, but vigorous efforts are undertaken to discover the cause of the tragedy in hope that future such events can be prevented.

At present, the annual fatality rate from breast cancer for women in America approximates the number of deaths in this hypothetical air disaster—each and every day! Yet unlike the approach undertaken by the NTSB to determine the cause and ultimately prevent future disasters, the focus in America regarding breast cancer remains fixated on treating the victims.

Hardly a day goes by that we are not encouraged by the announcement of some new form of breast cancer therapy. Unfortunately, even with our vast array of technical advancements today, one-third of breast cancer victims die from their disease. Remarkably, our cure rates for breast cancer remain about where they were some fifty years ago.

In light of these sobering statistics, it is imperative to recognize that our most well-respected medical journals have for decades been publishing high-caliber research studies indicating that preventive medicine may represent our most potent tool for dealing with breast cancer. Unlike the headlines made by so-called "breast cancer genes," risk factors over which we can exercise control and thereby help to prevent breast cancer, receive little fanfare.

The modern western medical paradigm places the healthcare consumer into an entirely passive role. We are conditioned to place our faith in medical technology and the products of the pharmaceutical industry in hope that "magic bullets" will treat the increasing number of maladies of modern society. This is exemplified by the recent attention given to a six year study of the drug Tamoxifen conducted by the National Cancer Institute. The study demonstrated a slight reduction of breast cancer risk in non-afflicted women taking this potentially dangerous drug. At the same time that Tamoxifen was making headlines, a landmark article was published in the *Journal of the American Medical Association* entitled, "Dual Effects of Weight and Weight Gain on Breast Cancer Risk" from the Harvard School of Public Health. Likely because this report did not advocate the use of a high-tech procedure or new pharmaceutical intervention, it received very little public attention. Nevertheless, this study did demonstrate a dramatic relationship between weight gain and breast cancer risk.

In a study reported in the prestigious *New England Journal of Medicine* it was found that in women 45 years or younger, regular exercise reduced breast cancer risk by an astounding 68%. A study published in the journal *Lancet* now provides almost irrefutable evidence of the link between a diet rich in phytoestrogen-containing foods like soy and lowered risk of breast cancer. A plethora of other studies have now made quite clear the relationship between other modifiable risk factors and the risk of breast cancer including pesticide exposure, alcohol consumption, and estrogen replacement therapy.

The Truth About Breast Cancer is about women choosing either to be passive and accept the one in eight risk of developing breast cancer and the subsequent one in three risk of dying from the disease, or being active and making those meaningful and profoundly therapeutic lifestyle changes which modern medicine has confirmed can have a major impact on reducing breast cancer risk.

David Perlmutter, M.D.
Naples, Florida
August, 1998

*"All truth goes through
three stages. First it is ridiculed.
Then it is violently opposed.
Finally, it is accepted
as self evident."*

Schopenhauer

ACKNOWLEDGEMENTS

Books are like movies in that while the author or director takes much of the credit for the project, a legion of people have worked "behind the scenes" on a variety of levels to bring the project to fruition. Whether in editorial, design, or production capacities, or simply by providing moral support, numerous people have assisted with this book. I am grateful for everyone who has become part of the process of delivering this message. While there is never enough space (or memory) to mention everyone, I will squeeze a few in here.

I am particularly grateful to David Perlmutter, M.D., a visionary healer who contributed the Foreword to this book. Special thanks goes to Neal Barnard, M.D., Keith Block, M.D., John McDougall, M.D., Helen Caldicott, M.D., John Robbins, and Michael A. Klaper, M.D., for their review of the material. I am grateful to Marion Moses, M.D. at the Pesticide Education Center for sharing her expertise on the health risks of pesticides. Deep appreciation goes to Paula Doubleday for her keen eye for design and production. Her interminable optimism and punctuality throughout the production process made an otherwise supreme challenge that much smoother. Jennifer Wengler, who worked with Paula on production, amazed me as she met each of the revisions with a perpetual certitude and cheerfulness. I thank Nancy Carleton for her editorial wisdom, Kathi Dunn for seeing my vision and gracing this book with its cover design, Connie Humphrey, personal trainer extrordinaire, for her kind referral, Nancy Gardner Heaven for sharing her expertise and enthusiasm for diagnostic thermography, and Ruth Heidrich, Ph.D. for sharing her insight as a breast cancer survivor, and for the tremendous inspiration she provides to women—and men, the world over.

Preface

In the spring of 1997, the National Institutes of Health (NIH) convened an expert panel to discuss whether to recommend regular mammograms for women in their forties. The panel's decision, which made headlines across the nation, was against recommending regular mammograms for women in their forties. Hours after this announcement, sharp criticism was directed at the panel of experts, and the already ardent debate over the appropriate frequency of mammograms escalated even further. Within a few days, the panel would announce the reversal of its decision.

Amidst this recent flurry in a long-running controversy, I had hoped that some attention might turn toward an area of less controversy: breast cancer prevention. As the shortcomings and risks associated with dependence upon mammography become increasingly apparent, prevention seems the only logical place to turn. For many, however, the idea that a woman might be able to influence her risk by making certain lifestyle choices is not even considered. After reading this book, I believe you will agree with me that prevention is not only worth considering but also the wisest place to focus our energy and our resources.

I became interested in breast cancer because of my family background. I was raised as a single son in a family of six women. Their concern and mine led me to do some research and to discover that, in fact, women can do much more to reduce the risk of breast cancer than perform self-exams and subject themselves to mammograms. Contrary to what women have been led to believe, a preponderance of evidence indicates that an array of strategies is available to help significantly reduce the risk for developing breast cancer.

Mainstream medicine has been quite vocal regarding breast cancer detection, but barely audible concerning prevention. In fact, the average woman knows very little about her own exposure to potential risks and her options for reducing the risks she can influence.

Almost daily there is some reference to breast cancer in the media. However, the kind of stories that seem to receive the most attention seem to be those that let people off the hook from taking personal responsibility. A prime example was the coverage of a claim that dietary fat has no relationship to risk of breast cancer. "Hooray!" you could almost here people exclaiming. For isn't that what everyone wants to hear? Did any of the journalists covering this story bother to take a look at the plethora of scientific papers that came before this single study — including studies that showed evidence that fat not only plays a role in the onset of breast cancer but also seriously impacts a patient's prognosis once the disease has been diagnosed? It is unlikely. Yet as you will see, dietary fat appears to be one of the primary controllable risk factors in breast cancer.

Recent polls indicate that few women genuinely understand or are aware of the risk factors for breast cancer to which they may be exposing themselves. Consequently, they have little knowledge about how they can help to prevent this disease. For example, a recent Opinion Research Corporation survey commissioned by the Physicians Committee for Responsible Medicine found that 80 percent of women are unaware of the potent relationship between their diet and breast cancer risk. Further, it was found that 55 percent of women polled considered performing self-examinations to be a preventive strategy, while 37 percent thought regular mammograms were preventive.[1]

As unfortunate as this is, it is not the fault of the women. After all, there has been considerable success in getting the word out about mammography, but, the question is, is it the right word? The lack of availability of preventive information for women and the overemphasis on detection strategies (mammography and self-exams) have resulted in women's thinking of detection strategies as preventive tools. A handful of other broad surveys confirm that women remain largely uninformed or misinformed about breast cancer and the strategies they can employ to reduce their risk.

The purpose of this book is to help you understand the risk factors identified by current research, clarify the areas where lifestyle changes can make a real difference, and put into practice strategies to prevent breast cancer. Part One of this book looks closely at the conventionally and not-so-conventionally accepted risk factors and examines how each factor may be playing a role in breast cancer risk. Part Two of this book outlines a comprehensive lifestyle plan specifying exactly what you can do to minimize your risk of breast cancer. Then, in the true spirit of prevention, we will look closely at what can be done to protect the next generation of women.

Along with recipes, dietary guidelines, and a comprehensive resource guide, the seven-step plan to prevent breast cancer is designed to give you the information that will enable you to begin at once to fortify your health and prevent not only breast cancer, but also a variety of other diseases that have similar risk factors to breast cancer, including heart disease, osteoporosis, hypertension, diabetes, and obesity.

Please understand that in light of the plethora of well-conducted studies that support the recommendations presented herein, no plan of action comes with a guarantee, and this book is no exception. However, after you have completed this book, I am confident that you will agree that the lifestyle recommendations made here are the most sensible and powerful choices a woman can make in the interest of prevention. Breast cancer is a multifactorial disease. This book will identify the risk factors affecting you, and help you make a transition toward a preventive lifestyle. I wish you well as you take your health into your own hands and empower yourself to reduce your risk of this deadly disease.

Joseph Keon, Ph.D.
Fall 1998

PART ONE

Risk Factors for Breast Cancer Every Woman Needs to Know

*"My own preference
is to tell people the truth...
and then let them decide
what would be their degree of compliance."*

Caldwell B. Esselstyn, Jr., M.D.

CHAPTER ONE

Breast Cancer: An Overview

WHAT IS CANCER?

Cancer occurs when there is unrestrained proliferation or growth of damaged cells anywhere in the body. Sites commonly affected include the lungs, breasts, stomach, colon, prostate, and uterus. The damage occurs to the proto-oncogene, a regulator gene that is found in DNA of the nucleus of every cell. Normally, the proto-oncogene can control cell growth and multiplication. However, once it has been damaged by way of a carcinogen, each offspring cell that proliferates will carry the same damaged oncogene. Often, the damaged cells no longer adequately perform their original tasks.

Most cancer is strongly related to environmental factors and lifestyle choices to which we expose ourselves.

While cancerous cells do not grow faster than healthy cells, they divide more often and live longer, and in doing so, they crowd out healthy, functional cells, competing with them for vital nutrients. This process can instigate a cascade of damage, including destruction of nerve pathways and bone. Cancer, whatever the type, is not necessarily an inevitable result of the aging process. Most cancer is strongly related to environmental factors and lifestyle choices to which we expose ourselves.

CURRENT PERSPECTIVES

Since 1950, breast cancer rates have been increasing at a rate of 1 percent per year.[2] In 1950, it was estimated that a woman had a 1 in 20 chance of being diagnosed with breast cancer in her lifetime. By 1976, the rates had climbed to 1 in 14. In 1982, estimates were 1 in 12; in 1989, 1 in 10. At the time of this writing, estimates are that 1 in 8 women will develop breast cancer in their lifetime, and a number of experts believe that by the turn of the century, it will be 1 in 6. Today, breast cancer is the leading cause of death for women between the ages of 35 and 50 in the U.S. **In 1998, 182,000 new cases will be diagnosed and 48,000 lives will be lost to the disease — another woman every 12 minutes — nearly as many Americans as were killed in the entire Vietnam War.** With each death from breast cancer, an average of 20 years of life have been lost, totaling 1 million U.S. life years annually. These staggering statistics are certain to continue until Americans take proactive stances and begin to practice preventive lifestyle choices.

The results of our current approach to cancer leave a great deal to be desired. Since former President Nixon declared "war on cancer" in 1977, little if any real progress has been made in stemming the incidence of cancer in the United States.* Our situation can be likened to mopping up water around an overflowing sink. Because we continuously expose ourselves to an increasing number of cancer-causing agents through

In medical school students hear little about the environmental and lifestyle-related causes of cancer and how we can stem the tide of disease through simple lifestyle choices.

toxic substances in our water, soil, air, and the foods we eat, we surely can't expect much progress. Before we can make any headway, we need to turn off the faucet — stop surrounding ourselves with carcinogens and stop following a high cancer risk lifestyle. Additionally, if corporations are permitted to continue to unleash thousands of pounds of toxic substances into our air, water, and soil annually, we should only expect things to worsen. Until the federal government takes a serious position and initiates policies that truly inform and protect citizens and the environment from ongoing toxification, we must expect an ongoing and increasing threat to human health.

---

*Kosary, C.L., et al., "SEER cancer statistics review," National Institutes of Health, Publication No. 96-2789; Devesa, Susan S., et al., "Recent cancer trends in the U.S.," *Journal of the National Cancer Institute* 87 (1995): 175-182.

THE PREVAILING MESSAGE

Hardly a week goes by without some newspaper or magazine article or radio or television talk show devoted to the subject of escalating breast cancer rates. Is all of this attention doing any good? In fact, the prevailing message has been pathetic. As an example, consider an article that made national headlines as I was completing this book. The article made reference to fish oils and suggested that women might be able to lower their risk of developing breast cancer if they took fish oil supplements. In the closing of the article, the head researcher interviewed was quoted as saying that "most breast cancer is due to reproductive history, genetics, and other factors over which women have little control."[3] The careless comment of the quoted researcher exemplifies the perpetuation of the myth that women are helpless in the face of this insidious disease. The point of my writing this book is to show you not only that this message is irresponsible, but also that a mountain of evidence from around the world indicates that it is not true.

Spending money on "magic bullet" studies, such as the fish oil study, diverts women's attention from the core issue — the causes of breast cancer. Doesn't it seem more sensible that we invest our resources to educate women and men about prevention? Suffice it to say that breast cancer is not caused by a lack of fish oils in the diet!

Another study that received a good deal of attention recently focused on the breast cancer drug called Tamoxifen. When the results of the study were released, the newspaper headlines read, "Drug Prevents Breast Cancer."

Researchers of the study suggested that, based on their investigation, the drug could be given to women who are considered "at high risk," as a form of prevention. Within a few days, the very people who put Tamoxifen on the map condemned the study and the suggestion that the drug be prescribed to healthy women in hopes of preventing future breast cancer.*A major concern was that the study had been abruptly ended 14 months ahead of schedule. Longer running studies of Tamoxifen were conducted by researchers at the European Institute of Oncology in Milan and The Royal Marsden Hospital in London. Neither of these studies supports the use of Tamoxifen as a "preventive drug" in cancer-free women. Dr. Trevor Powles, leader of the British study states, "I have grave concern about the wide spread use of [Tamoxifen] in healthy women."

---

*New York Times, April 8, 1998; Associated Press, July 10, 1998.

Tamoxifen is called a Selective Estrogen-Receptor-Modulator (SERM). The drug works by selectively blocking estrogen in some tissues while behaving like estrogen in others. It was discovered some 40 years ago, and has for the last 20 years been prescribed to "high risk" women who have already been treated for breast cancer in hopes that it will reduce the likelihood of recurrence. Do to the media attention the drug has received, many women with whom I have spoken are anxious to know if they are candidates for taking the drug. It is therefore imperative that women know about the darker side of Tamoxifen.

Very serious potential risks are posed by Tamoxifen, including damage to the retina and corneal opacities, a 700 percent increased risk of developing potentially fatal blood clots, and serious risk of hepatitis and liver and uterine cancer.

Tamoxifen is an indisputable carcinogen. In 1995, the California State-appointed Carcinogen Identification Committee, a nine–member expert panel lead by University of Southern California's Dr. Thomas Mack, confirmed Tamoxifen "unequivocally carcinogenic" to both humans and animals. A seventeen–member panel of the International Agency for Research on Cancer of the World Health Organization formally confirmed Tamoxifen a carcinogen in February 1996.

While the most recent study of Tamoxifen did report a 45 percent reduction in the incidence of breast cancer for the women who took the drug over the short run, it is still not clear if the drug is in fact preventing breast cancer or simply delaying the time in which cancer appears. Side effects of the drug were noted in this study as follows. In women in the study there were also 33 cases of endometrial cancer (14 in the placebo group), 17 cases of potentially fatal blood clots in the lung (6 in the placebo group), and 30 cases of dangerous clots in major veins (19 in the placebo group). The study showed that Tamoxifen doubled the risk of uterine cancer.

Many of the papers that reported the Tamoxifen study failed to point out a disturbing conflict of interest associated with the drug maker. Zeneca Group PLC of the U.K., the manufacturer of Tamoxifen, with some $470 million in annual sales of the drug,* also happens to market a cancer-causing herbicide called acetochlor, whose annual sales are estimated at $300 million.[4] How does one justify being in the market of both an agent that *causes* cancer, and another, its purported cure?

---

*If Tamoxifen is prescribed for the 29 million American women the National Cancer Institute estimates are at "high risk," annual sales of the drug could climb to $7.5 billion.

Since the World Health Organization estimates that up to 80 percent of the cancers we see in humans today are a consequence of diet choices and exposure to environmental carcinogens[5] (cancer-causing chemicals), and the American Institute for Cancer Research estimates that between 30 and 50 percent of all breast cancer can be prevented through a healthful diet and regular exercise, we will all benefit when research removes its fixation from diagnosing and treating cancer and focuses on preventing it in the first place. Doing so will save not only millions of lives but also billions of dollars in health-care costs.

Why don't we focus more resources on preventing disease? Because we live in a society whose medical infrastructure has been built around the treatment and management of disease. Consider that the National Cancer Institute, whose annual budget is approximately $2 billion dollars, devotes a paltry 5 percent to the area of prevention. Medical schools teach their students about intervening with disease using sophisticated and expensive technology, but students hear little about the environmental and lifestyle-related causes of cancer and how we can stem the tide of disease through simple lifestyle choices. After all, they are not paying many thousands of dollars to learn about nutrition. It is astonishing that after the United States surgeon general stated that approximately 70 percent of the diseases that afflict Americans are directly related to their dietary choices,[6] only 30 of the 125 medical schools in America require their students take a single nutrition course.[7] Once doctors begin to practice, opening up to preventive strategies becomes even more difficult. Insurance companies do not reimburse physicians for nutritional counseling. Deviating from the protocol of colleagues risks disapproval and ostracism, so it appears better to practice medicine as the others do. Of course, greater numbers of conventionally trained physicians are branching out and beginning to incorporate more alternative approaches to achieving and maintaining wellness. A handful of physicians have even achieved celebrity status doing so. However, these mavericks are not free of detractors, and some have been ruthlessly insulted as "quacks," "nuts," and "charlatans." The resistance to preventive health care is still very strong.

While we have made enormous strides in terms of understanding the causes of cancer and ways to prevent it, the information is not reaching the public in a form that genuinely facilitates lifestyle changes. Most Americans are dangerously uninformed about their own health and what they can do to protect it, and consequently, they do not reap the benefits of this knowledge.

The Truth About Breast Cancer will help you understand the ways you may be at risk for breast cancer, and how you can take this knowledge and use it to make real-life changes that reduce your risk and increase your level of health, your overall well-being, and your peace of mind.

CHAPTER TWO

Who Is at Risk?

Everyone is at risk for breast cancer, both male and female, although the disease affects many more women than men.* Breast cancer is a multifactorial disease, and numerous factors contribute to its risk, including the following conventionally accepted risk factors: sex, race, family history, early menarche, late menopause, late or no pregnancy, not breast-feeding, long-term estrogen replacement therapy, alcohol consumption, body size, and the less considered factors: exposure to cigarette smoke, breast implants, radiation, stress, exposure to environmental toxic substances, and diet.

CONVENTIONALLY ACCEPTED RISK FACTORS

Sex

Obviously, being female confers a much higher risk of breast cancer than being male. For every 100 cases of breast cancer in women, there is 1 case in men. Many of the additional risk factors, such as those relating to menarche, menopause, pregnancy, and breast-feeding relate to women as opposed to men.

Race

Caucasian women are more at risk for breast cancer than women from racial groups with darker skin. While women obviously cannot alter their racial background, women with higher indicators for risk can pay even greater attention to minimizing other risk factors.

---

*Breast cancer strikes about 1,000 men each year in the U.S., and rates are increasing. While this book is written for women, much of the preventive lifestyle information applies to men as well. The same guidelines will also reduce the risk of prostate cancer in men, which currently has an incidence similar to that of breast cancer in women.

Family History/Heredity

Another risk factor for breast cancer is family history. A good deal of attention has been given to the breast cancer genes BRCA 1 (stands for "breast cancer 1") and BRCA 2. BRCA 1 is found in those families with a history of breast cancer and ovarian cancer. BRCA 2 is found in families where there is a history of both male and female breast cancer. A third gene, called TSG101, has also attracted considerable attention. TSG101 is a gene that normally suppresses tumor development. Studies have shown that in some women with breast cancer

Studies have shown that women who reach menarche before age 13 have a 4.2 times higher risk of developing breast cancer later in life.

this gene is missing or damaged.* While genetic heritage is certainly important, in reality only about 6 percent of today's breast cancer incidence can be attributed to a genetic predisposition. Carrying the BRCA 1 or BRCA 2 gene is not a death sentence; it by no means guarantees that you will develop breast cancer. Carrying either gene is a disadvantage and should be seen as all the more reason to make lifestyle choices that we know can reduce risk and increase protection.

A woman whose mother had breast cancer has an elevated risk herself, about double if her mother's cancer occurred before the age of 40. More important seems to be whether or not cancer occurred in a sibling. If a woman's sister developed breast cancer, she has 2.5 times the risk of developing it herself than if her sister were cancer-free. Interestingly, if you have a brother who is diagnosed with prostate cancer, your chance of developing breast cancer increases four times.

Early Menarche

The age at which a woman first menstruates is a risk factor for breast cancer for a simple reason. The earlier a woman begins having periods, the more periods she will have over her lifetime, and consequently the more estrogen she will be exposed to.

---

*Limin, Li, et al., *Cell* 88 (1997):143-154.

Studies have shown that women who reach menarche before age 13 have a 4.2 times higher risk of developing breast cancer later in life. A woman who enters puberty at age 12 will be exposed to five additional years of menstruation, and consequently five more years of heightened exposure to estrogen. This exposure will be taking place at a time when the breast tissue is particularly susceptible.

Your first reaction might be, "How can I influence the onset of my first period? Isn't that up to my genes?" It appears that a woman *can* have a great deal of influence over when periods begin. While this is not a risk factor adults can address for themselves, it is one that parents can consider for their offspring (see Chapter 18 on protecting the next generation). Children today are maturing at a much faster rate than ever before, and experts are pointing their finger at diet and at exposure to industrial chemicals.[8] A good deal of attention is being focused on the role of dietary fat. Dietary fat and overall energy intake influence the production of hormones. The more fat consumed, the higher the hormone levels become. Elevated hormone levels can instigate physical maturation that may not have occurred in a more natural state. Certain industrial chemicals are also being investigated because of their potential to mimic or interfere with hormones in the body, and thereby possibly stimulate physical changes.

At the turn of the 20th century, the average age of menarche was 17 years. It is now 12.5 years of age. A recent study found that a significant number of girls are showing signs of puberty by age 7. Even more disturbing, the study found that 1 percent of girls in the U.S. today are exhibiting physical changes such as breast development and pubic hair by age 3![9] In many countries that were previously protected by their traditionally low-fat diets but where the high-fat Western diet is slowly being adopted, the same trend can be seen. For instance, in Japan, fat intake has traditionally been much lower than in the U.S. However, with the relatively recent introduction of hundreds of fast-food restaurants, fat intake is rising sharply and the age of menarche is falling. The average age at which girls enter puberty has dropped from 15.2 to 12.5 in only the past four decades in Japan.[10] Yet according to T. Colin Campbell, Cornell University biochemist and director of the China Health Study, in rural China, where fat consumption is still among the lowest in the world, girls reach puberty between 15 and 19 years of age.

It has been estimated that risk of breast cancer can be reduced by 10 percent to 20 percent for every year that menarche is delayed.[11]

Late Menopause

Late menopause is also a risk factor for breast cancer. Menopause that occurs after the age of 55 is considered late. When the risk associated with late menopause is taken into account, perhaps this time of life will begin to be more welcome. Obviously, the longer a woman continues to ovulate, the greater her lifetime exposure to estrogen. Therefore, the later menopause occurs, the higher the risk may be.

Women who begin menstruating earlier in life tend to experience a late menopause by four to five years. When we consider the combined effect of early menarche and late menopause, we are looking at about eight to ten years of additional exposure to heightened estrogen levels.

Remember, because of the fat-induced elevation in hormone levels, women who follow a high-fat diet increase their chances of a later menopause.

Estimates are that women who experience menopause before age 45 reduce their risk of breast cancer risk to half that of women who continue to menstruate into their mid-fifties and later.

Late or No Pregnancy

Another risk factor for breast cancer in women is pregnancy later in life or not at all. Each month, the cells of the breasts go through a maturation process. The process is not completed unless there is a full-term pregnancy. Without pregnancy, the cells are left "immature," and as a result, their DNA is less stable and is vulnerable to carcinogenesis. With pregnancy and lactation, the cells are stabilized, and risk is reduced. Therefore, the shorter the period between menarche and first pregnancy, the lower the risk. Late pregnancy is considered to be one that occurs after age 30. Risk is reduced further if the first pregnancy occurs before the age of 20. While earlier and multiple pregnancies reduce one risk factor for breast cancer, there are clearly multiple considerations that go into a woman's decision to bear a child and when to do so, so it is not necessarily wise for pregnancy to be used as a "prevention strategy." For some women, reducing their risk in this area is simply not a realistic option.

Not Breast-Feeding

Not only does North America have the distinction of having some of the highest rates of breast cancer in the world, it also has the peculiarity of one of the lowest rates of breast–feeding in the world.[12]

Not breast-feeding is also considered a risk factor for breast cancer. Studies have shown that risk is reduced for women who breast-feed for at least four months, and the longer they breast–feed, the lower their risk, particularly before the age of 20.[13] The latest recommendation from the American Academy of Pediatrics is that women should breast-feed their infants for at least a year. Not only does breast–feeding reduce the risk of breast cancer, but also, research has confirmed a reduction in the risk of ovarian cancer. For the baby, breast milk is a near miracle food that bestows incredible health benefits, including lowered risk of allergies, infections, diarrhea, skin rash, and pneumonia.

Unfortunately, some 38 percent of American mothers never even try to breast–feed, and a mere 15 percent nurse their baby for a full year.[14] Again, breast-feeding as a way of reducing risk for breast cancer is an option that is not available to all women. The reduced risk for this disease, however, is another reason for women who bear children to commit themselves to breast-feeding if at all possible.

Long-Term Estrogen-Replacement Therapy

Controversy continues over the risks and benefits associated with long-term use of estrogen-replacement therapy (ERT) and hormone-replacement therapy (HRT). Numerous studies have reported inconsistent results with regard to the effectiveness of ERT and HRT in reducing menopausal and post-menopausal symptoms. Effective or not, there is sufficient evidence that such therapy poses a breast cancer risk.[15] Additionally, estrogen replacement therapy increases breast tissue density which may in turn obscure mammographic images and lead to a false diagnosis.*

ERT has been justified largely based upon the assertion that it will reduce risk of osteoporosis and heart disease. Most women are unaware of the fact that both diseases are largely preventable through lifestyle choices, which may preclude the need for debate over such therapy. Further, there is evidence that natural progesterone creams, and even soy foods, may offer a safer alternative for menopausal symptoms such as hot flashes. Hormone-replacement therapy is examined more fully in Chapter 8.

Alcohol Consumption

It has been shown repeatedly that alcohol raises estrogen levels in the body and increases the risk of breast cancer in both premenopausal and post-menopausal women.[16] Researchers at the National Institute of Environmental

---

*Laya, M.B., et al., *Radiology* 196 (1996):433-7.

Health Sciences found that one drink a day was sufficient to increase breast cancer risk by 10 percent. Two drinks a day increased risk by 20 percent when compared to women who drank no alcohol.[17] A meta-analysis* of 16 studies conducted by researchers at Harvard University suggested that two drinks a day may increase risk by as much as 70 percent when compared to nondrinkers.[18]

There are several reasons alcohol may increase risk. First, as mentioned, alcohol increases estrogen levels.[19] Estrogen is metabolized by way of two paths, one short and the other long. The short path is considered safer because this is how non-cancer-promoting estrogens, such as plant estrogens, are transported. The long path is taken by environmental estrogens from industrial chemicals, by estrogens in hormone therapy, and estradiol, the estrogen that seems to be the breast cancer promoter. Alcohol may temporarily inhibit the short route for estrogens to reach receptor sites and, as a consequence, leave receptor sites open for the more dangerous type of estrogen. Additionally, some alcoholic beverages contain known carcinogens, and alcohol also impairs the immune system, which plays a role in keeping cancerous cells in check.[20]

Those who were most overweight had a risk almost twofold of dying after diagnosis than those with the lowest levels of body fat.

Body Size

Body size is also a risk factor for breast cancer. In America, we seem to celebrate heavy babies and tall children as an indication of robust health to follow. I have often heard a mother boasting about her child's rank in national height percentiles. Unfortunately, research has shown that adults who were heavy babies are at greater risk for a number of degenerative diseases, including cancer.[21]

Taller women (over 5 feet 6 inches) tend to have a greater risk for breast cancer than women who are 5 feet 3 inches or less. Being overweight also confers greater risk.[22] A study from the Harvard School of Public Health found that women who gained 22 to 44 pounds since the age of 18 had a 60 percent increase in risk. Those who gained more than 44 pounds in that period were at double the risk.[23]

---

*A meta-analysis involves the pooling of data from preceding studies. This process creates one large study in which important findings, not discovered in smaller single studies, may be revealed.

Once breast cancer has been diagnosed, a woman's prognosis is worse if she is overweight.[24] In the Iowa Women's Health Study, which examined mortality rates for over 690 women diagnosed with unilateral breast cancer, it was found that those who were most overweight had a risk almost twofold of dying after diagnosis than those with the lowest levels of body fat.[25] Comparison studies in Japan found that obese women were more likely to die within five years of diagnosis than their thinner counterparts.

While women cannot change their height and basic body frame, a commitment to a good diet and exercise, which lead to a leaner body, can make a difference in reducing this risk factor.

LESS CONSIDERED RISK FACTORS

Many of the risk factors outlined to this point are largely out of our control. There is little you can do about your height today, or about your genetic heritage, or for that matter, the age at which menarche occurred for you. It is important to note that **while the conventionally accepted risk factors for breast cancer (heredity, late or no pregnancy, early menarche, body size, not breast–feeding, late menopause, etc.) all play a synergistic role in risk, the reality is that in 70 percent of all cases of breast cancer, these factors do not play a role.**

The factors that follow here are those which are seldom considered in the conventional discourse about breast cancer. Make no mistake, however, that each plays a very important role.

Exposure to Cigarette Smoke

Smoking has been linked to a variety of diseases, not the least of which is breast cancer. Even the nonsmoker is at great risk. Women who are exposed to secondhand smoke have a 300 percent increased risk of breast cancer. Secondhand smoke contains larger quantities than firsthand smoke (because the filter reduces them) of the cancer-causing ingredients aromatic amines, including 4-aminobiphenyl and B-naphthylamine.[26] An American Cancer Society study of one million women found that smoking as a teenager is particularly hazardous because the chemicals in cigarette smoke may have an imprinting effect on developing breast tissue, setting the stage for breast cancer decades later in life.

Breast Implants

Breast implants and the possible risks they pose are an extremely controversial topic. Despite the fact that there are thousands of pending lawsuits against the makers of implants, the number of breast augmentation surgeries has increased 275 percent in just the last 5 years, according to the American Society of Plastic and Reconstructive Surgeons.

Currently, it is estimated that over 1 million American women have breast implants, the majority of which are for the purpose of enhancement in otherwise healthy women. While no direct relationship between implants and elevated risk for breast cancer has been demonstrated thus far, there are a number of concerns of which women should be aware.

Although there is yet definitive proof, some studies suggest that implants may elevate risk of an autoimmune reaction in which the body turns on itself, attacking healthy cells and possibly leading to the development of diseases such as arthritis, scleroderma, and lupus.*

Another potential risk is posed by older silicon implants. While there is no conclusive evidence about the risks of silicone in humans, studies with animals are not reassuring. Animals injected with silicone develop aggressive malignant tumors. Further risk may be posed by the polyurethane foam with which some implants are coated. The coating contains a compound called 2,4-toluene diisocyanate, the carcinogenicity of which has been confirmed by the Environmental Protection Agency and the Federal National Toxicology Program. Further risk may be posed by Ethylene oxide, a sterilizing agent that is often used on implants before they are inserted. While the risk posed to humans from Ethylene oxide exposure is unclear, the International Agency for Research on Cancer has confirmed that it instigates tumors in animals.

A concern that we are most certain of is the tendency of implants to obscure a significant portion of imageable breast tissue in mammography. Because of the impaired imaging, there is an increased risk of missing an existing cancer that might otherwise have been detectable.

Radiation

Medical radiation is another risk factor for breast cancer. Aside from environmental, accidental, or catastrophic exposure to radiation, the primary source of radiation exposure is medical. Many X-ray technicians are fond of saying "It's only a small dose" to their patients who question exposure to medical radiation. While the dose of medical radiation of a typical X-ray

---

*Lancet 340 (1992):1304-1307; Archives of Internal Medicine 153 (1993):2638-2644; Journal of Investigative Surgery 9 (1996): 1-12; Clinical Rheumatology 14 (1995):667-672; Toxicology and Industrial Health 10 (1994):149-154.

(or mammogram) has been reduced over the years, this does not eliminate its danger. The fact is that medical radiation is a human carcinogen *at any dose* because exposure to it can result in cellular mutations. This is one reason for the abundance of controversy surrounding the use of regular mammogram screenings. We will look at the subject of radiation exposure through mammography in detail in Chapter 3.

Stress

Another risk factor for breast cancer is stress. We all know that stressful life events can take a toll on our health. Yet the toll is more than simple fatigue. Chronic stress can seriously debilitate the body's immune system, and therefore the body's ability to defend itself from disease. Most of us think of the immune system protecting us from opportunistic diseases, such as bacterial infections and viruses, but the immune system also plays an important role in preventing the development of cancer. Individuals who respond poorly to stress show a marked reduction in natural killer (NK) cell activity — cells whose job it is to patrol the body for and eliminate cancer cells before they proliferate. Researchers using a standardized stress test and measuring blood samples have found that those who report the most traumatic stresses in their lives showed the greatest reduction in NK cells. Conversely, researchers have found that when individuals are taught stress reduction strategies, NK cell activity can increase by as much as 30 percent.[27] In Chapter 7, we will look in more detail at stress as a factor in disease, and in Part Two, you will learn stress reduction strategies that can become a regular part of your life.

Exposure to Environmental Toxic Substances

As we will explore further in Chapter 6, exposure to environmental toxic substances is a major risk factor for breast cancer. From the water we drink, to the foods we eat, to the air we breathe, each year we are exposed to a greater number of toxic chemicals. Currently, researchers are looking at a variety of chemicals not only for their carcinogenicity, but also, for their potential to disrupt normal hormone activity in the body, and possibly heighten risk of breast cancer. Lifestyle changes can reduce exposure to many of these toxic substances, but reducing exposure to others will take awakening the awareness of the general population, and motivating citizens to pressure governmental leaders to change policies that permit the proliferation of toxic chemicals from industrial operations.

Diet

I list diet last because I am of the researched opinion that, along with exposure to toxic chemicals and medical radiation, it is the strongest risk factor involved in the development of breast cancer. In fact, over a decade ago, the National Research Council published a report in which it proposed that diet was the most significant factor in the epidemic of breast cancer. Surprisingly, a recent survey found that 80 percent of women polled had no idea that their dietary choices could influence their risk of developing breast cancer.

Diet is one risk factor that most all women in the U.S. share. Diet may be the most powerful risk factor we can control, one which can mitigate the effects of many of the toxic substances to which we may be exposed on a regular basis, as well as the other risk factors for breast cancer that lie outside our control. The choices we make each day can influence our health for years to come, and all of us make dietary choices at least three times a day.

The preponderance of research linking diet and cancer is so overwhelming that I have devoted Chapters 4 and 5 to discussing it further, and in Part Two, I will go into detail about how preventive dietary changes can reduce your risk of breast cancer. There is so much you can do, if you choose, to prevent breast cancer.

CHAPTER THREE

The Uncertainties of Mammography

As the previously mentioned survey indicated, the role of mammography is largely misunderstood. The effectiveness and risks associated with mammography are also largely a mystery to women. Mammography is the primary and often only thing women think of when considering their risk of breast cancer. I feel it is essential that this tool and its shortcomings be defined before you read about any of the other risk factors in this book. A quotation from *The Lancet* states: "The benefit [of mammography] is marginal, the harm caused is substantial, and the costs incurred are enormous." After completing this chapter, perhaps you will concur. This chapter should make it abundantly clear that prevention, and not the hope of "early detection," is our best strategy in contending with breast cancer.

"Women have been led to believe that there is this tool out there that's going to save our lives. But it's just not true"

The National Cancer Institute (NCI) estimates that $2 billion is spent annually for breast cancer screening in the U.S. General Electric sells over $100 million a year in mammography machines.[28] The National Cancer Institute estimates that there are 14,000 mammography machines installed in the U.S., two to three times more than is required for current mammographic needs. Each year some 24 million mammograms are performed.

There is no question that the use of mammography in the U.S. is big business. There is a question, however, about the quality and safety of the service that is provided for this staggering sum of money.

The year 1997 was a volatile year for mammography. In a period of just three months, an expert panel assembled by the National Institutes of Health (NIH) stated that it felt there was no reason to recommend mammography screening to women in their forties. Its advice was that women in this age group should "decide for themselves." At the same time, the American Cancer Society (ACS) was recommending that women in their forties have a mammogram every year. This recommendation was an increase from its previous recommendation of "every one to two years." At the same time, the National Cancer Institute (NCI) was recommending that if a woman is at "average risk" of developing breast cancer, she should have mammograms every one to two years.

Very quickly, the NIH's recommendation that women in their forties avoid mammography drew sharp criticism from the medical community, and subsequently the NIH reversed its recommendation. This galvanized the already contentious debate over the effectiveness and safety of mammography screening.

Why is there such controversy over this diagnostic tool? Here are a few concerns that every woman needs to be aware of before making a decision about whether to have regular mammograms, and if so, how often and at what age.

THE MYTH OF MAMMOGRAPHY IN BREAST CANCER PREVENTION

Do you remember the non sequitur "Early detection is your best prevention"? This popular slogan appeared in ads on the radio, on television, and in print to promote reliance upon mammography. In fact, public health organizations and magazine articles assured women that mammography was their best chance at preventing breast cancer.[29] Although the slogan is seldom heard anymore, the flawed logic persists in the minds of millions of women. As the previously mentioned survey by the Physicians Committee for Responsible Medicine indicated, 37 percent of women surveyed believe that mammograms are a preventive tool.

The Chant of "Regular Mammograms"

If you ask the average woman what she should do to prevent breast cancer, often her reply will be that she should get regular mammograms and perform self-exams. Women have been hearing for years that mammograms and self-exams are important in preventing breast cancer. For the most part, this is the only message women have heard. Unfortunately, it is dead wrong. When I give a presentation about breast cancer, the very first thing I say is that mammograms do not prevent breast cancer. They never have, and they never will.

Many women have acquired a false sense of confidence from the chronic chant of "regular mammograms and self-exams." Responsible health-care practitioners don't ever directly promise that mammograms prevent breast cancer. However, simply by the fact that the campaign is so strong in the absence of any other strategy, diagnostics have been misconstrued as preventive. The tremendous emphasis placed on mammography without offering any useful prevention information has diverted women's attention from the truly preventive strategies they could be practicing. As one woman said to me, "What's there to do? You get your mammogram and just hope you're not the next one."

A good deal of the ongoing debate about recommending regular mammography screening pertains to its ability to provide advanced notice of an existing cancer. The logic is that if one detects the cancer early enough, eradication will be more likely.

"Women have been led to believe that there is this tool out there that's going to save our lives. But it's just not true," says Fran Visco of the National Breast Cancer Coalition. Studies of mammography suggest women should heed Ms. Visco's words.

DEFINING "EARLY DETECTION"

For a cancer in the breast to be detected by our current mammography equipment, about 30 cell divisions must have taken place.[30] These divisions occur at a rate of between 25 and 200 days, with the average taking about 110 days. At the rate of 110 days, the tumor might be detected in nine years (110 days x 30 divisions). That means the cancer has been growing in the body for nearly a decade — sufficient time for an additional problem to arise. This problem is called metastasis. In metastasis, cancerous cells may break away from the original tumor, and use the blood vessels or the lymphatic system to travel to and infiltrate other organs of the body. As the cancer colonizes other organs, successful eradication becomes very unlikely. In fact, metastatic cancer is what kills. Obviously, even if earlier detection increases survival rates, it is clearly preferable to prevent breast cancer in the first place.

Another drawback to mammography as a diagnostic tool is that, as the National Cancer Institute confirms, **the technology fails to detect tumors in as many as 25 percent of cases for women in their forties**. The error rate is even higher in premenopausal women due to greater tissue density. In 70 to 80 percent of positive readings, a follow-up biopsy shows the patient to be cancer-free.[31] According to a *Lancet* study, the rate of false positives may be as high as 93 percent.[32] In other words, there are many false positives. With those false positives comes an untold degree of undue fear and anxiety—even after it has been determined cancer is not present. In one study, 26 percent of women continued to experience anxiety a full three months after it had been determined they were cancer-free.*

Some research has indicated that mammography can actually increase the risk of metastases, through the compulsory compression of the breast during screening. If cancer cells are present during this compulsory compression, the cells can be pushed in a way that they may spread out to other parts of the body.[33]

THE DANGER OF MEDICAL RADIATION

Mammograms pose another problem: They emit ionizing radiation, a risk factor for cancer itself. This fact receives curiously little attention. Because of the focused way in which the radiation is delivered during a mammogram, mammography poses a particular risk for breast cancer.[34] If you have ever asked a radiologist administering an X-ray about the safety of the procedure, you likely heard the all-too-common retort, "It's only a very small dose." Others are fond of saying, "You'll receive more radiation on a flight to Paris

Because of the focused way in which the radiation is delivered during a mammogram, mammography poses a particular risk for breast cancer.

*Annals of Internal Medicine 114 (1991):657.

than from this X-ray." Both of these responses need to be addressed. While a single film today may expose a woman to only a fraction of the radiation used in the past, we simply cannot ignore the fact that ionizing radiation is a human carcinogen at any dose. This means that a cellular mutation could occur with a single exposure or after 20 or more exposures. We simply cannot know. Because of the latent period of carcinogenesis, a cancer that has been initiated by medical radiation may not manifest for anywhere from 5 to 50 years. Furthermore, each dose of radiation we receive is cumulative — more time in between exposures does not lessen the risk.

A flight from the U.S. to Paris, France, might expose a passenger to 5 millirads of cosmic radiation; however, this smaller dose is dispersed to the entire body. A mammogram focuses radiation on one area of the body. An average mammogram will result in an exposure of about 300 millirads (a millirad is one-thousandth of a rad) of radiation for each image taken. However, if there is a suspicious area in the first films, she may be exposed to 10 or more follow-up x-rays, with a total dose of radiation of 3,000 millirads or more. Because of this very real risk, it seems humane and ethical that patients be exposed to medical radiation only when absolutely necessary, and then only after being informed of the associated risk.

In 1963, John William Gofman, M.D., professor emeritus of molecular and cell biology at the University of California at Berkeley established the Biomedical Research Division for the Livermore National Laboratory, where he actively researched the relationship between chromosomal abnormalities and cancer. Having received the Right Livelihood Award in 1992 for his work to expose the health effects of low-level radiation, today, through his work with the Committee for Nuclear Responsibility (CNR), Dr. Gofman is one of the most outspoken advocates of the responsible use of radiation.

In his book *Preventing Breast Cancer*, [35] Gofman states his belief that, in conjunction with other factors, 75 percent of all breast cancer today is the consequence of previous radiation exposure, derived primarily from medical sources, such as X-rays, from infancy through adulthood. Dr. Gofman recognizes as valid the numerous other risk factors associated with breast cancer, but believes that in the absence of prior radiation exposure, such factors may not play as large a role.

Considering the degree to which diagnostic and therapeutic radiation has been used, the likelihood of its role in today's cancers becomes quite clear.

THE PROLIFERATION OF MEDICAL RADIATION

Consider that it was once a practice to perform pelvimetry (pelvic X-rays) and placentography (X-rays of the placenta) to ascertain whether a woman was going to be able to give birth vaginally. Radiation therapy was used to treat post-partum mastitis, a condition in which the breasts become infected. Fluoroscopy (use of an X-ray device) was commonly employed to evaluate tuberculosis. Radiation therapy was used to treat bronchial asthma, and in the treatment of pneumonia and hyperthyroidism. Monitoring the progress of scoliosis (curvature of the spine) required ongoing X-ray exams. For a period of time, fluoroscopy in shoe stores was common to ascertain proper shoe size. This procedure not only exposed the customer, but also, because of radiation scatter, nearby children, their parents, the shoe fitter, and other bystanders in the store who were within a 25-foot radius of the fluoroscopy machine. There was a time when beauty shop personnel administered radiation to treat hypertrichosis (unwanted body hair on the face, breasts, and other areas), and dermatologists found the technology effective in treating skin disorders such as eczema (in some cases of the breast), dermatitis, and psoriasis. Many women, therefore, have already been exposed repeatedly to radiation, a major risk factor for breast cancer.

Haphazard Administration

As can be seen, historically we have relied upon X-ray technology to a greater degree than could be considered safe. In conjunction with this, numerous surveys over the years have shown an alarming incidence of faulty X-ray machines, untrained operators, and patient overdosing. An FDA study showed that, depending on where the X-ray was administered, the dose of radiation from a chest X-ray could vary one hundred-fold. Surveys of mammography facilities are equally discouraging. One found that of 319 facilities nationwide, only 71 percent regularly monitored the dose of radiation emitted. In another survey of 96 mammography units in the state of Michigan, 8 exceeded the "acceptable" dose of radiation, and 36 had other problems.[36] In a survey that was printed in the *Wall Street Journal*, state officials estimated that 15 to 50 percent of machines inspected did not meet patient safety requirements, and that as many as 20 percent of administrators did not have formal training in radiology.

In the same article, Dr. Robert Quillin, director of the Ohio Radiological Health Program, was questioned about a device called a collimator. The collimator is used to direct the beam of an X-ray. The wider a collimator is set, the more broadly the beam is broadcast, and the greater the degree of superfluous exposure, or what technicians call "scatter." When a collimator is set properly, the beam is directed to the most specific area being filmed, limiting unnecessary exposure. Dr. Quillin indicated that it would not be unusual to find collimators wide open in random inspections of machines. The result, he says, is X-ray exposure "from your knees to the top of your head."[37] These drawbacks apply to mammography as well as to other forms of X-ray technology.

DIAGNOSTIC ALTERNATIVES

You now may be asking, "Okay, so what am I supposed to do now?" With the well-established shortcomings and risk associated with mammography, there is a growing interest in alternative imaging technologies. One promising technique is digital mammography. While it still uses X-rays, with the assistance of advanced digital enhancement, the images are sharply improved, and can be enhanced on a screen utilizing special software which may reduce the need for follow-up images to be taken, necessitating further exposure. There are other diagnostic techniques as well, each with certain drawbacks but none of which emit X-rays, including ultrasound, magnetic resonance imaging (MRI), Anti-Malignin Antibody Screening (AMAS), and thermography. These diagnostic alternatives are worth considering either in place of or as an adjunct to conventional mammography.

Diagnostic Ultrasound

Ultrasound uses high-frequency sound waves to create a "map" of parts of the body. The technology can be a useful adjunct tool. For instance, the FDA has approved this technology to assist in evaluating a suspicious area appearing in a mammogram. Researchers agree that rather than performing a potentially unnecessary biopsy, that is both painful and leaves scar tissue that can be misinterpreted in future breast imaging, ultrasound can often be used to better assess the area of concern.[38] Clinical investigators have suggested that up to 40 percent of current biopsies could be avoided when ultrasound is used to distinguish between benign and malignant lesions. While it is far from perfect (it is unable to detect lesions that are less than one centimeter in size), in a recent study conducted by radiologist Dr. Thomas Kolb, ultrasound used in conjunction with mammograms detected 195 cancers that mammograms alone failed to detect.[39]

Consider that 700,000 women undergo a breast biopsy annually in the U.S. Nearly 80 percent of the biopsied specimens turn out to be benign (non-cancerous). The biopsy procedure results in both internal and external scarring, which may complicate accurate interpretation of future breast imaging. There is, of course, also the emotional trauma a woman faces between the time when a biopsy is ordered and when the results are delivered.

Because it helps differentiate between benign and malignant tumors, ultrasound, used in conjunction with either mammograms or physical exams, could reduce the necessity for such biopsies by as much as 40 percent, according to clinical investigators.

Magnetic Resonance Imaging (MRI)

Magnetic resonance imagery utilizes magnetic fields to create a differentiated image of body tissues that are injected with a contrast dye that concentrates in cancer cells. The technology is particularly useful for detecting tumors in the more dense breast tissue of premenopausal women and in women with implants. Although the technology is sometimes used in place of biopsy after a suspicious finding, it fails to distinguish between benign and malignant lesions. The current cost (about $800) also makes mass screenings using MRI technology too costly. MRI may become more commonplace in the near future, and this, of course, will help to bring the cost down.

Diagnostic Thermography

A thermograph is essentially a picture of heat energy emissions (natural infrared or electromagnetic energy) from the body that have been converted to electronic video signals that appear on a video screen. Cancerous cells, which grow in an unregulated fashion, generate more heat than healthy cells, and so tumors tend to be "hotter" when viewed with thermography. A cancerous area also exhibits hypervascularity or greater blood flow to the area. An essential part of diagnostic thermography is to make a comparison of images taken before and after the patient's hands are exposed to cold water. Normally, the cold water will result in constriction of blood vessels and a body temperature drop of about 0.25° C. When cancer is present, the body temperature may stay the same or even go up, as blood flow increases to the afflicted area, and more energy is emitted in the thermograph.

Free of radiation, thermography is a highly sensitive tool that is noninvasive and pain-free because it does not require breast compression. In fact, no device or person touches the body during the exam, nor do any rays of any kind enter the body. Using thermography, it may be possible to detect a cancer as much as five years before a mammogram.[40] Further, according to thermography expert Philip Hoekstra, Ph.D., who has personally screened over 50,000 women using thermograms, the technology is between 86% and 96% accurate in revealing a cancer in premenopausal women. Dr. Hoekstra says that when there is an error, in almost all cases it is a false positive, meaning while the screening indicated a potential cancer, none was actually present. Obviously this is more desirable than a false negative.

Another advantage of thermography is that, unlike mammography, in which image quality diminishes with breast density, thermograms read well regardless of tissue density, and therefore are particularly useful for younger women with imaging needs. A shortcoming of thermography is that it is unable to show a mass for biopsy purposes. However, if it detects a suspicious zone, it may then warrant a mammogram for biopsy purposes. Thermography is therefore well worth considering as an alternative to mammography for screening purposes. (See Resources).

Anti-Malignin Antibody Screen (AMAS)*

Another alternative to mammography is an anti-malignin antibody screen (AMAS). In the presence of cancer, the body produces defense molecules known as antibodies. One of the antibodies that is present when a cancer exists is called anti-malignin, a protein whose job is to attack the inner–most layer of a cancer cell.

Sam Bogoch, M.D., identified this cancer marker after many years of research, and states that his laboratory's AMAS test is 95 percent accurate on the first test and 99 percent accurate when repeated, in detecting anti-malignin. The exception is in very advanced stages of cancer when the anti-malignin antibody is *One of the antibodies that is present when a cancer exists is called anti-malignin, a protein whose job is to attack the inner–most layer of a cancer cell.* virtually eliminated. According to Dr. Bogoch, the presence of tumors as small as 1 to 10 millimeters can be detected by the AMAS test, something a mammogram cannot do.[41]

---

*The AMAS test is intended for detecting early stage cancers. It is not appropriate for detecting advanced stage cancers in which there is severe immune suppression and the antimalignin antibody is virtually eliminated.

Since a mammogram alone cannot determine whether a suspicious area is a malignancy or benign, rather than perform a biopsy or lumpectomy, the AMAS test could be performed to obtain a reliable diagnosis. The AMAS test is an FDA-approved and patented procedure that is available to anyone under the care of a licensed physician who can order the test. The test costs around $135, with a follow-up cost of approximately $85. For further information about AMAS, please see the Resources section.

THE BOTTOM LINE

In this chapter, we have explored some of the drawbacks to mammography, as well as some of the alternatives. The bottom line is that each woman has to decide for herself whether or not to get a mammogram, and then how often. The key is that you have a choice. It should be kept in mind that most breast cancers (almost 90 percent) are in fact discovered by physical exam. For example, a survey conducted by the San Francisco organization Breast Cancer Action found that of 226 women with breast cancer who were interviewed, 44 percent discovered the cancer through self-exam, 37 percent through mammograms, and 8 percent through physician's exam.

In 1997, when the National Institutes of Health convened its expert panel to determine whether to continue to recommend mammography for women in their forties, one panel member, Duke University's Dr. Donald H. Bening, stated that at best 1.5 percent of women in their forties receive any benefit from annual mammograms. One study found that more than half of the breast cancers treated in premenopausal women were not detectable by mammography.[42] Another study analyzing the results of the most prudent studies on mammography indicates that screening women under the age of 50 is of little value.[43] As mentioned before, this is primarily due to greater breast tissue density in premenopausal women which makes imaging difficult. Based upon current evidence, the U.S. Preventive Service Task Force, American College of Physicians, International Union Against Breast Cancer, Canadian Task Force on Periodic Health Examinations, and the European Group for Breast Cancer Screening are all in alignment with the recommendation that screening mammography not begin before the age of 50. In fact, much of the rest of the world does not recommend screening mammograms before age 50. This is not to say that if you or your health–care practitioner find a suspicious lump a mammogram shouldn't be performed.

When you do have a mammogram, be sure that your exam takes place in a dedicated mammography clinic, meaning that mammography is what is done there exclusively. Also be sure that the clinic's equipment is certified by the American College of Radiology. Make sure that the person administering the mammogram is a mammography specialist (if it's a dedicated center, he or she should be) who holds a state license to perform mammography and that your film is interpreted by a certified radiologist. You may even wish to confirm that the clinic's machine has been calibrated in the last year, and, if you are comfortable doing so, you may request a report on the clinic's annual rate of false positives and false negatives.

The timing of a mammogram may also be an important consideration. As mentioned earlier, tissue density is a primary reason why mammographic images are so poor in younger women. The greater the density the less likely an accurate image will be rendered. A number of studies have shown that breast tissue density varies considerably throughout the menstrual cycle.* The most recent study on this subject, published in the *Journal of the National Cancer Institute*, found that among 2,591 pre-menopausal women aged 40-49, breast tissue density was much greater during the second half (the luteal phase) of their menstrual cycle than during the first half (the follicular phase). Therefore, it seems wise that should a mammogram be required the procedure be planned for sometime in the first two weeks of the menstrual cycle.

The role of prudent monthly self-exams and annual clinical exams can not be underestimated, particularly if there is a history of breast cancer in your family. If you are not comfortable with or don't feel proficient performing self-exams, seek out self-exam training from a qualified physician or a program such as Mammacare (see Resources).

Remember, while self-exams and other diagnostic tools can help detect breast cancer, which can and does save lives, they cannot and do not prevent breast cancer in the first place. Nevertheless, there are many steps you can take to reduce your risk of breast cancer. In Part Two of this book, you will learn strategies that are truly preventive.

---

*Baines, C.J., et al., *Cancer* 80 (1997):720-4; Bjarnson, G.A., *Lancet* 347 (1996):345-6; Hrushesky, W.J., *International Journal of Cancer* 59 (1994):151.

CHAPTER FOUR

The Dietary Connection

My earlier book, *Whole Health*, devoted a large section to demonstrating the relationship between diet and disease. Most people have no idea that the most prevalent diseases in America (cancer, heart disease, Type II diabetes, osteoporosis, hypertension, obesity, and so forth) are very closely correlated with dietary choices. As you will see in this chapter, breast cancer is no exception. The food choices we make can reduce or elevate the risk for breast cancer as well as other life-threatening diseases.

Despite enormous amounts of evidence demonstrating the crucial role of diet, there has been a great tendency to play down the

Over 20 years ago, researchers at the National Cancer Institute showed the strong relationship between animal fat consumption and breast cancer risk.

significance of this factor. In fact, studies that downplay the role of diet seem to get the biggest headlines. As John McDougall, M.D. says, "People love to hear good news about bad habits," and Americans have some really bad dietary habits.

THE ROLE OF FAT

While there are several dietary factors that increase the risk of breast cancer, the most important is fat. Let's see why this much-maligned nutrient is back on trial again.

An abundance of scientific papers confirm the role of dietary fat as a significant risk factor for breast cancer.[44] Classic experimental work conducted in the 1950s showed that dietary fat can encourage tumor growth in animals,[45] and other research has shown specifically that dietary fat enhances mammary tumor growth in animals.[46] Substantial epidemiological and experimental evidence in humans and animals has shown that a strong relationship exists between the daily intake of dietary fat and the incidence of breast cancer.[47]

While a more recent well-publicized study, the Harvard Nurses Study, suggested that there was no relationship between fat and breast cancer risk, the study had shortcomings. Not the least of these was a failure to include subjects consuming 20 percent or less of their calories as fat. Comparing subjects who eat an ultra-high-fat diet with those who eat a high-fat diet is not going to prove much of anything. It is like comparing those who smoke two packs of cigarettes a day with those who smoke a pack and a half a day. The overwhelming evidence is that as fat intake increases, so does the risk of breast cancer.[48]

What About the 30 Percent Fat Guideline?

The prevailing guidelines from the U.S. government and a variety of public health organizations suggest that one should aim for a diet that derives 30 percent of its calories from fat. Unfortunately, **no scientific evidence exists to support such a recommendation.** As hard to believe as this may seem, no scientific evidence was used to arrive at such a figure. Indeed, it is an arbitrary number that most experts believed was "achievable." The executive summary of the National Academy of Sciences 1982 report states: **"The scientific data do not provide a strong basis for establishing fat intake at precisely 30 percent of total calories. Indeed, the data could be used to justify an even greater reduction."**[49] There is a good amount of scientific evidence that a diet that derives 30 percent of its calories from fat offers no protection against cancer.[50] In fact, studies have shown that in terms of cancer incidence, there is no difference between a diet of 40 percent and one of 30 percent of calories as fat. Evidence suggests that for real protection, dietary fat intake needs to be reduced to 20 percent of calories or less.[51]

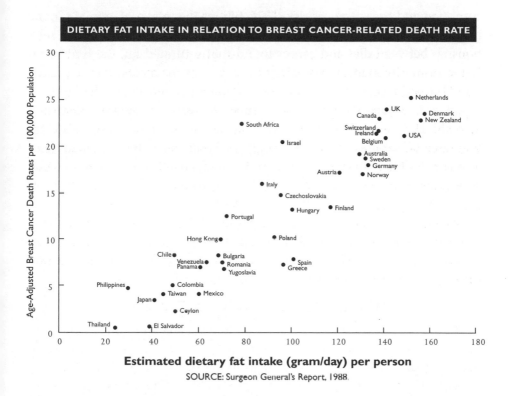

DIETARY FAT INTAKE IN RELATION TO BREAST CANCER-RELATED DEATH RATE

Estimated dietary fat intake (gram/day) per person

SOURCE: Surgeon General's Report, 1988.

Invariably, countries with the highest intake of fat (particularly animal fat) show a correspondingly high incidence of breast cancer. This is also true of male breast cancer. Men living in West Germany consume an enormous quantity of dietary fat — almost 50 percent of their daily calories — and West Germany has the distinction of having the highest incidence of male breast cancer. Conversely, those countries with the lowest intake of fat have only a fraction of the breast cancer seen in the United States.

Further, in studies with animals where tumors had occurred spontaneously or had been chemically induced, researchers found that the more fat the animal consumed, the more rapidly the cancer grew. Metastasis (the spread of the cancer) to lymph nodes and lungs was more likely and more severe in the animals fed the higher–fat diet.[52]

Animal vs. Plant Fat

Animal fat, prevalent in the Western diet, seems to pose a greater risk than fat derived from plants. Over 20 years ago, researchers at the National Cancer Institute showed the strong relationship between animal fat consumption and breast cancer risk.[53] The higher the intake of animal fat, the higher the incidence of breast cancer. A recent study examining the relationship between diet and cancer found that saturated fat, the type of fat found primarily in meat and dairy products, was the most accurate predictor of breast cancer risk. The more saturated fat women ate, the higher their risk.[54] **A U.S.-Japan Cooperative Cancer Research Program researcher, Takeshi Hirayama, has documented a 380 percent increased risk for women who eat meat once a day compared with those who eat meat once a week.**[55] Other studies have corroborated this finding.[56] In general, Americans, both men and women, eat an enormous amount of meat. Their diets are centered upon meat, and it is not uncommon for three or more meals a day to include beef, pork or poultry. In fact, **according to the U.S. Department of Agriculture, the average American will consume 21 cows, 14 sheep, 12 hogs, 900 chickens, and 1,000 pounds of fowl and seafood during the course of his or her lifetime.**

Migration Studies: Following the Trail of Fat

Rates of breast cancer have traditionally been relatively low in Japan. In fact, research has shown that the incidence of breast cancer is six to eight times higher in the United States than in countries in Asia.[57] Historically, between 10 and 20 percent of the calories in the Japanese diet came from fat.[58] That is changing today with the proliferation of American fast-food chains and Western eating habits. In fact, the introduction of the high-fat, low-fiber American eating style has shown a concomitant increase in disease, including cancer, in Japan.[59] During the period 1970-1985, breast cancer incidence has more than doubled in Japan.[60] The older generation, which has largely maintained the traditional diet, is now in some cases outliving its children, who are succumbing to the consequences of the Western high-fat, low-fiber diet: cancer and heart disease.

Even so, breast cancer rates are still far lower in Japan than in the U.S. At one time, it was thought that there was something unique to Japanese women, something other than controllable lifestyle factors playing a role in their lower risk. Migration studies suggest otherwise.[61] It is telling that **when Japanese, Chinese, and Filipino women migrate to America and adopt Western lifestyle patterns (including the high-fat, low-fiber Western diet), they assume the risk rates of American women.** Not only does their mortality rate begin to match that of American women, but their offspring display an even higher rate.[62]

Fat and Hormone Levels

Dietary fat may be a contributing risk factor for several reasons. The first is its influence on estrogen levels. As a woman's dietary fat intake rises, so do levels of circulating estrogen. This in turn may heighten the exposure of breast tissue to estrogen, a known risk factor for breast cancer.

Conversely, when dietary fat levels are reduced, estrogen levels drop.[63] An important study conducted by researchers at the University of California, Los Angeles showed that by following a very low-fat diet, the estrogen (specifically estradiol) and prolactin (another hormone that is elevated in breast cancer patients) levels of female subjects were halved in only three weeks![64] Other studies have shown similar results.

A high fat intake usually leads to the accumulation of more body fat. The more body fat you have, the more estrogen you will produce. This is because fat cells, with the assistance of the enzyme aromatase, convert androgens (a male hormone occurring in both sexes) to estrogens in women.

A vegetarian diet is by nature lower in total fat than an omnivorous diet. A vegan diet (one that excludes all forms of animal products — meat, fish, poultry, eggs, milk, cheese, etc.) is, of course, even lower in total fat. One study found that premenopausal vegetarians had 23 percent lower levels of circulating estrogens than omnivores. Postmenopausal study participants who followed a vegan diet were found to have estrogen levels up to 40 percent lower than matched omnivores.[65]

Body Fat and Prognosis After Detection

Women with a greater degree of body fat have a worse prognosis after diagnosis with breast cancer.[66] Women who consume the most fat also have a worse prognosis after detection. In the Iowa Women's Health Study, researchers looked at the relative risk of dying after breast cancer diagnosis in relation to dietary fat intake and other variables. They found that the women who consumed the greatest amount of fat had a risk of dying more than twice that of the women who consumed the least amount of dietary fat.[67] Another study found that for every 1,000 grams of fat consumed monthly by patients, the relative risk of death increased 44 percent.[68]

Some animal studies have indicated that once cancer has been established, a high-fat diet increases the likelihood that the cancer will metastasize (spread) to other areas, such as the lymph nodes and lungs.

High Fat Intake and Mammograms

If you are going to expose yourself to mammography, you would obviously wish to have the best, most accurate film produced, thereby eliminating the need for further mammograms and minimizing cumulative exposure to ionizing radiation. (For a further discussion of mammography, please see Chapter 3).

As a woman's intake of dietary fat increases, so does the density of her breast tissue.[69] When breast tissue is dense, it becomes more difficult to "read" a mammogram. This is why the false negative rate tends to be higher in premenopausal women — their breast tissue is more dense at this time in life.

Greater breast density is associated with increased risk of breast cancer.[70] In an important study published recently in the *Journal of the National Cancer Institute*, researchers found that women with a very high breast density have a fivefold increased risk of breast cancer.[71] Fortunately, this is another area that women can influence. The good news is that research conducted at the Ontario Cancer Institute in Canada showed that **a low-fat diet can reduce breast density and thereby not only lower risk of disease but also improve the ability for mammography to render a clear image.**[72]

Fat and Toxic Chemicals

Dietary fat — specifically animal fat — is also a source of concentrated drug and chemical residues such as hormones, fungicides, and pesticides, many of which are known human carcinogens. When farm animals are given feed that is contaminated with pesticide chemicals, the chemicals ultimately find their way to the animal's fat, where they bioaccumulate. When that animal is eventually eaten by humans (for example, as a steak, hamburger, or chicken breast), whatever payload of chemicals has accumulated in its body then bioaccumulates in human body fat, the breast being one prime area. The enormous amount of animal flesh that the average American consumes over a lifetime offers a tremendous opportunity for a person to consume and bioaccumulate whatever hazardous products have found their way into the bodies of these animals.

It is well known that women with higher concentrations of such chemicals in their body have a higher incidence of breast cancer. In fact, **researchers at Mt. Sinai Medical Center in New York have found that malignant (cancerous) breast tissue samples contain 50 percent to 60** percent higher concentrations of pesticide residues than healthy tissue.[73] Finnish researchers found that women who had high levels of the pesticide hexochlorocyclohexane had a ten times increased risk of developing breast cancer.[74]

Another terribly sad indicator of the degree to which we are being exposed to toxic chemicals is mother's milk. Numerous studies have been conducted to look at the types of chemicals that are accumulating in human tissue, and breast milk is an excellent indicator. The findings are frightening.[75] Today's mother's milk samples have revealed residues of over 100 toxic chemicals, some known human carcinogens. The pesticide residue levels in these samples alone exceed the standards set for cow's milk. In fact, it has been said that **mother's milk, due to its toxicity, would be subject to ban by the FDA if it were bottled for sale on supermarket shelves**. The physical and psychological benefits infants receive from breast-feeding, and the nutrients found in human milk as opposed to soy or cow's milk, still make breast-feeding a healthier choice for both mother and child, but the presence of toxic chemicals in breast milk serves as a warning sign of the way dietary fats concentrate toxic chemicals in the food chain.

Clearly, dietary fat is a major risk factor for breast cancer, and one that lies within women's power to reduce. **Research involving international comparisons, time-trend analysis, migration studies and case control studies suggest that if current levels of dietary fat in the U.S. were halved, breast cancer risk could be reduced by about 250 percent**.[76] You will learn exactly how to make that reduction in Chapters 19 through 22.

Two additional dietary factors that play an important role in preventing not only breast cancer but also numerous additional diseases are dietary fiber and important plant compounds called phytochemicals. Research also shows that a high-fat diet that is low in fiber is particularly dangerous.[77] In Part Two, you'll learn more about the importance of fiber and phytochemicals and how to include more of them in your diet while reducing fat intake.

CHAPTER FIVE

High-Risk Foods

So far we have seen clearly that a strong correlation exists between the incidence of breast cancer and dietary fat intake. More specifically, we have seen that the association between fat intake and risk is greater when the fat is derived from animal products and when the consumption of fiber is low. This chapter will look at a few specific foods that pose a risk when the diet emphasizes them.

Dr. Roland Phillips of Loma Linda University's Department of Biostatistics and Epidemiology has proposed that a diet that is based upon plant foods may well allow the body's immune system to operate at more optimal levels simply because of the absence of foreign animal proteins. Dr. Phillips hypothesizes that a body that is not in a state of constant hypervigilance contending with other foreign proteins, such as bovine proteins, is better suited to be patrolling for and eliminating the early replicants of tumor cells.

Casein, a protein found in cow's milk, has also been implicated as a cancer promoter.

Aside from the risk of consuming foreign proteins, which can elicit numerous unwanted health effects, a number of other potential risks are associated with a diet that is centered upon animal products.

DAIRY PRODUCTS

There is no reason whatsoever for humans to consume the milk of another species, and a preponderance of scientific evidence suggests they should not do so. The ancient Greek physician Hippocrates noted that cow's milk could cause skin rash and gastrointestinal problems. We know this well today, yet we keep hearing the same message: Drink more milk; eat more yogurt; have another slice of cheese. Unfortunately, a skin rash is the least of the potential problems posed by consuming cow's milk.

Contrary to the favorable image generated by clever television commercials and print advertisements, a substantial body of scientific evidence suggests that cow's milk is not the health food that many people have come to believe. Cow's milk and products made from it are one of the leading causes of allergy. Dairy products also tend to be high in cholesterol and saturated fat, excesses of which have been linked with atherosclerosis and heart disease, and can cause, or are associated with a higher risk of, a variety of symptoms, including diarrhea,[78] abdominal pain, iron deficiency anemia,[79] gas, eczema, arthritis,[80] bloating, migraine headaches,[81] asthma,[82] runny nose, lower I.Q.,[83] sudden infant death syndrome (SIDS),[84] juvenile diabetes,[85] acne, fatigue, ovarian cancer,[86] immune dysfunction, and an elevated risk of osteoporosis.[87] Dairy products almost always contain antibiotic residues,[88] which can elicit allergic responses in some people, and pesticide, and synthetic hormone residues,[89] some of which have been linked to cancer in humans.

The Allergy Problem

Food allergies are quite pervasive, but because there is often a delay in the onset of symptoms, few people attribute their condition to the foods they have eaten. Dairy products are no exception. Cow's milk contains a variety of different bovine proteins to which an individual may have an allergic response. It is not until individuals entirely eliminate an offending food from their diet that they see and feel the association between their health and that food.

Lactose Intolerance

Mother's milk plays a big part in providing the protein and calcium that are so critical during the early stages of human development. Yet after infancy, milk is no longer a necessity because other foods have become palatable. **Humans are the only animals that continue to "nurse" after infancy, and it is much to our detriment.** In fact, many people are incapable of properly digesting cow's milk after the infancy stage because of the lack of a digestive enzyme called lactase. Lactase is necessary to break down the disaccharide sugar in milk called lactose. When lactase is present, lactose is broken down into two monosaccharide sugars, glucose and galactose. In most cases, the body progressively stops manufacturing this enzyme by age four, although it may continue to do so in small amounts.

Those whose bodies no longer produce this digestive enzyme have difficulty digesting cow's milk and other dairy products. The undigested lactose moves to the large intestine, where it is attacked by bacteria that convert the undigested sugar to gas and lactic acid. The result may be a number of side effects, including bloating, diarrhea, gas, and abdominal pain. **Some 50 million Americans may experience this intestinal distress from consuming dairy products but may or may not make the association between their pain and what they have just eaten.**[90] The highest prevalence of lactose intolerance is among Thais (90 percent), Japanese (85 percent), Greenland Eskimos (80 percent), Arabs (78 percent), African Americans (70 percent), Israeli Jews (58 percent), and Native Americans (50 percent).

The Cancer Connection

The consequence of consuming lactose in dairy products may be much more serious for women. A recent study has shown a correlation between the consumption of dairy products and breast cancer risk.[91] **Researchers at the Harvard School of Public Health found an increased risk of ovarian cancer in women with a high intake of dairy products, particularly yogurt and cottage cheese.** In fact, the highest rates of ovarian cancer are seen in countries where the greatest quantity of dairy foods is consumed.[92] Casein, a protein found in cow's milk, has also been implicated as a cancer promoter. Dairy product consumption has also been associated with recurrent vaginitis, menstrual cramps, fibroids, and increased pain from endometriosis.[93]

Cow's milk and products produced from it in regions where nuclear power plants operate pose a unique hazard. Nuclear power plants are regularly releasing into the air, water, and soil, cancer-causing nuclear fission products such as the deadly radioactive isotope strontium-90. When these emissions land on the grass and in the water that dairy cattle feed on, they end up in the milk the animal produces. Areas in which high levels of strontium-90 have been detected in the food show a correspondingly high incidence of breast cancer.[94]

Bovine Growth Hormone (BGH) and Breast Cancer

Like meat, milk carries a risk of exposure to hormones, pesticides, antibiotics, and other chemicals that may end up in the milk supply. In 1993 came the publicity regarding the biosynthetic (genetically engineered) milk hormone called BGH, or BST. BGH was developed for the purpose of making dairy cows produce greater yields of milk — a seemingly superfluous goal considering the enormous surplus of dairy products produced in the U.S. annually. BGH appears to work, not only at increasing milk yields, but also, the risk of serious disease in both cows and humans.*

Dr. Richard Burroughs, a veterinarian who spent half his 13-year career working for the Food and Drug Administration studying the effects of bovine hormone use in cows, says, "The very first data I saw come in showed that it [BGH] increased reproductive and udder infections in cows." These sick

The Food and Drug Administration's (FDA) Total Diet Study found pesticides in 70 percent of cheese samples tested.

cows, with a condition known as mastitis, must then be treated with sulfa drugs and numerous other antibiotics routinely fed to sick dairy cows.[96]

Seemingly unbothered by this finding, the FDA approved BGH as a hormone supplement for dairy cows. Rather than move into uncharted waters, Europe placed a moratorium on BGH until the year 2000. Recent findings indicate that the wait was a wise decision.

While studies had already shown that BGH induced cancer in mice, in 1996, Dr. Samuel Epstein, professor of environmental toxicology at the University of Illinois, Chicago, reported that BGH may be associated with an elevated risk for breast cancer in humans.[97] Recently, this assertion has been corroborated by a number of studies which suggest that BGH-tainted dairy products are a risk factor for breast cancer. The most recent study, reported in *The Lancet*, shows a 700 percent increased risk of breast cancer among pre menopausal women with the highest levels of IGF-1 in their blood.[98] IGF-1 is a natural hormone found in humans and cows. When cows are injected with BGH, their levels of IGF-1 are elevated, and eventually pass into their milk, which is then drunk by humans, thereby raising human levels of IGF-1.

---

*For a detailed look at BGH and dairy products, please see Robert Cohen's book, *Milk: The Deadly Poison* (Englewood Cliffs; Argus Publishing, 1998)

Dr. Epstein rightly points out that "**with the active complicity of the FDA, the entire nation is currently being subjected to an experiment involving large-scale adulteration of an age-old dietary staple by a poorly characterized and unlabeled biotechnology product**. Disturbingly, this experiment benefits only a very small segment of the agrochemical industry while providing no matching benefits to consumers. Even more disturbingly, it poses major potential public health risks for the entire U.S. population."

The Diabetes Connection

Cow's milk may also be responsible for eliciting an autoimmune response that leads to diabetes mellitus in susceptible children.[95] Type I (or insulin-dependent) diabetes can severely compromise the quality of life and result in premature death. The disease is caused by the inability of the damaged pancreas to produce insulin. Studies of a portion of one of the proteins in cow's milk, bovine serum albumin (BSA), have indicated that BSA may instigate an autoimmune response that leads to the destruction of the beta cells of the pancreas.

The Pesticide Problem

As previously stated, animal products are the primary sources of pesticide residues in the American diet. Finding a conventionally produced milk or milk product today that is free of pesticide residues is an increasing challenge. For example, the Food and Drug Administration's (FDA) Total Diet Study found pesticides in 70 percent of cheese samples tested.[99] In the same study, thirty-two different pesticide residues (including vinclozolin, a known endocrine-disrupting chemical), were found in sixteen samples of fruit-flavored yogurt.

The Antibiotic Problem

The *Wall Street Journal* conducted an independent investigation of the safety of milk, and its study revealed antibiotic drug residues in 40 percent of the milk samples taken from ten major American cities.* Contrary to what one would hope, public awareness hasn't mitigated the problem. In a recent FDA Journal, **investigators reported finding 16 illegal drug residues in the cows at an Oregon dairy farm, including streptomycin, neomycin, and gentmycin.**[100] It is not reassuring to know that the FDA only tests for a

---

*The *Wall Street Journal*, December 29, 1989.

handful of over 80 drugs currently used. The fact is that dairy cattle are raised in conditions that are likely to promote disease and necessitate the use of antibiotics to keep the cows producing for the farmers.

The Leukemia Problem

A little-known fact is that, on average, 80 percent of the American dairy herds are infected with bovine leukemia.[101] Can the disease cross species and infect humans? Certainly not if the milk has been properly pasteurized. Is there a chance that unpasteurized milk can reach the public? Such a mistake has already occurred.* Suffice it to say that no one needs leukemic cow's milk on their corn flakes.

The Protein Problem and Bones

Cow's milk is excessively high in protein, and excess protein intake is one of the major causes of osteoporosis. When we consume excess animal protein, our blood may become too acidic in nature, and to buffer this acidity, the body will draw upon alkaline minerals including calcium, from the bones. Today's trend toward low-fat milk exacerbates this problem. In the interest of lowering the high-fat content of cow's milk, the proportion of protein has been raised.

Building strong bones and keeping them fortified over time is the primary justification for consuming dairy products such as milk and cheese. Unfortunately, the scientific and epidemiological evidence to support this assertion is nowhere to be found. In fact, one study, sponsored by the dairy industry itself, showed just the opposite — that women who supplemented their diet with a few extra glasses of milk a day were in a negative calcium balance (they were losing more calcium than they were keeping) when the study was completed. This is just one of many studies that challenge the age-old myth that humans need to drink the milk of another species in order to maintain bone integrity. The recent Harvard Nurses Study, which included over 77,000 women, found that women who drank three or more glasses of milk a day had no reduced risk of hip or arm fractures during a 12-year follow-up period. Moreover, **the women who drank three glasses of milk a day had a higher incidence of fractures than women who drank little or no milk at all.**[102]

One of the most telling discoveries in the area of bone health research came from Cornell University researcher Dr. T. Colin Campbell, who heads the Study on Diet, Nutrition and Disease in the People's Republic of China.

---

*For a further look at the bovine leukemia problem, please see breast surgeon Dr. Robert M. Kradjian's letter at http://www.earthsave.bc.ca/impact/articles/health/milk_letter.html

Considered to be the "Grand Prix" of such studies, the data collected have taught us a great deal about lifestyle and risk of disease, including osteoporosis. Dr. Campbell says, **"Ironically, osteoporosis tends to occur in countries where calcium intake is highest and most of it comes from protein-rich dairy products."** This includes the United States, Canada, Northwest Europe, Australia, and New Zealand. The study found that the average daily intake of calcium in China is 544 mg, and osteoporosis is quite rare. This is compared to the average daily intake of calcium in the U.S., which is 1,143 mg, and osteoporosis is near epidemic in the U.S.

The answer to this apparent riddle is quite simple. While calcium is essential to bone health, and dairy products contain calcium, with the calcium comes a payload of animal protein, phosphorus, and sodium, all of which, in excess, can make calcium more difficult for the body to absorb and retain. In fact, no other dietary factor links so tightly with calcium losses and risk of bone fracture than excessive protein intake. Yet the excess protein in the American diet comes not just from the milk, yogurt and cheese, but from the large quantities of beef, chicken, pork, and eggs in the average American diet. It is encouraging to know that when one reduces the intake of animal protein, calcium losses can be significantly reduced. **In a study reported in the *American Journal of Clinical Nutrition*, it was found that simply eliminating animal protein from the diet resulted in a reduction of calcium losses by more than 50 percent.**[103] An excellent model supporting this finding is the native Inuit population. Because they subsist primarily on fish, seal, and whale meat, and consequently consume an inordinate number of bones, their calcium intake is one of the highest in the world — over 2,500 mg a day. With such a calcium intake, one might expect these people to have particularly strong bones. Unfortunately, this is not the case. Because of their meat-centered diet, the Inuits also have one of the highest intakes of animal protein in the world, and consequently, they have the distinction of having the highest incidence of hip fractures worldwide.

MEAT

One of the primary sources of saturated fat and cholesterol in the American diet, meat is a major influence in the development of many diseases, including breast cancer. A debate continues over whether or not humans were ever intended to eat a meat-centered diet. World famous paleoanthropologist Dr. Richard Leakey cautions that "We are not carnivores and never have been carnivores, and that should be remembered." Although many humans eat an omnivorous diet, it is interesting to note the differences between true carnivores and humans. If one looks at the evolutionary history of human beings, it is clear that, until relatively recently, we have primarily been herbivores, or plant eaters. In support of this fact, our teeth are mostly flat for grinding plant foods, unlike the teeth of carnivores, or meat eaters, which are pointed and sharp, designed for effectively piercing and tearing flesh. Even our clawless hands are useless for this purpose. True carnivores also have the seemingly unlimited capacity for processing, assimilating, and ridding themselves of the massive amounts of cholesterol they consume each day. Consequently, they do not suffer from hardening of the arteries. The human body has only a limited capacity for contending with large amounts of cholesterol and saturated fat, and, consequently, excesses lead to disease. Our intestinal tract is different from that of carnivores. True carnivores have very short digestive tracts best suited for rapid elimination of meat. Herbivores, on the other hand, like humans, have long intestinal tracts that are suited for digesting plant foods. However, even with these clear physiological differences, we humans manage to eat meat, and we pay a heavy price for it.

Meat is a protein-heavy and phosphorus-rich source of food, excesses of both of which are linked strongly with osteoporosis and kidney disease.

The Protein Problem

The fat that is contained in animal products has long been implicated in promoting cancer, but more recently, it appears that excess protein itself may elevate risk.[104] Head of the China Project, Dr. T. Colin Campbell says findings indicate that animal proteins play a significant role in carcinogenesis, and that when consumed beyond the body's need, it appears the protein excess encourages precancerous lesions and tumors to grow.

Other researchers have found that after instigating a cancer in animals by way of a known carcinogen, a high-protein diet caused their animal's cancer to develop quite rapidly. Conversely, when the animal was fed a low-protein diet, their cancer slowed markedly and was even extinguished. In the same experiment it was found that protein excesses from plants did not promote a cancer nearly to the degree that excesses from animal products did.

The Iron Problem

Meat contains excessive levels of iron, which acts as an oxidant, leading to the production of free radicals. Free radicals not only cause cellular damage and expedite the aging process of tissues, but also are linked to cancer and birth defects. Iron can oxidize cholesterol, making it easier to clog up arteries and thereby heightening risk of heart disease, as well.

The Fiber Problem

Another major drawback of meat consumption is that meat is totally lacking in fiber, which is very important in controlling weight, preventing colon cancer, and stimulating immune function, not to mention in helping to maintain hormonal balance by facilitating the excretion of estrogens.

The Pesticide Problem

Meat is often tainted with chemical pesticides, and fertilizers, many of which have been shown to be carcinogenic to humans. In fact, beef contains higher residues of chemical herbicides than any other U.S. food. For a detailed look at pesticides in food, see Chapter 10.

The Hormone Problem

Hormones with which cows and hogs are routinely treated to rapidly increase their size, often end up tainting the meat. **Current estimates are that 90 percent of chickens, 80 percent of veal calves and hogs, and more than half of all beef cattle are given hormones as either implants or hormone-supplemented feed.** Roy Hertz, a hormonal cancer specialist and former director of endocrinology of the National Cancer Institute, explains that these added hormones pose serious risk, particularly for hormonally sensitive tissue such as breast tissue. Just how dangerous they are is illustrated in the following:

A little-known fact is that, on average, 80 percent of the American dairy herds are infected with bovine leukemia.

A horrendous tragedy has resulted from people consuming hormone-tainted meat on more than a few occasions. There have been instances in numerous countries around the world in which **children as young as four years old experienced breast development, uterine enlargement, body hair, and even menstruation, all as a consequence of eating meat that was contaminated with large amounts of hormones.** A wish to avoid such a tragedy is precisely why the European Economic Community has banned the importation of beef from North America for over a decade. Keep in mind that the USDA does not test the U.S. meat supply for hormone residues.

The Antibiotic Problem

Livestock are also fed enormous quantities of subtherapeutic antibiotic drugs, residues of which remain in the meat for the consumer. U.S. livestock receive half of all antibiotics produced annually.[105] This is helping to breed greater antibiotic-resistant strains of bacteria. While nobody should be unwittingly consuming antibiotics in their food, some individuals are exquisitely sensitive to such drugs and can suffer allergic reactions to them, and even death. Furthermore, antibiotics, particularly tetracycline, inhibit calcium absorption, elevating the risk of osteoporosis.

More Than You Bargained For

Most recently, it has been learned that drug and antibiotic residues are not the only risks one faces with meat consumption. In October 1997, Physicians Committee for Responsible Medicine held a press conference to make known the morbid practice of feeding chicken feces to cattle. Its report, which was published in *Preventive Medicine*, revealed that **in 1994 18 percent of poultry producers in Arkansas fed some 1,000 tons of chicken feces to cattle — feces that may contain E. coli bacteria, Salmonella, Campylobacter, parasites, drugs, chemical contaminants, and varying levels of arsenic, cadmium, and lead.**[106] This appears to be an excellent way to pass antibiotic-resistant bacteria from one animal to another. Additionally, cattle feed in the U.S. is known to contain a variety of additives, including poultry feathers, ground newspaper, plastic pellets, sewer sludge, sheep and cattle remains, cement dust, cardboard, and sawdust.[107]

Bacterial Contamination

As if these were not sufficient reasons to exclude meat from your diet, there is also the problem of an increasing incidence of bacteria poisoning from meat consumption.

Bacterial contamination has become an increasingly serious problem in the U.S.[108] Names like E. coli, Listeria, Campylobacter, and Salmonella have become all too familiar in recent years. E. coli 0157:H7 (commonly referred to as E. coli) is an extremely virulent strain of bacteria that can cause severe illness and even death when present in very small amounts. In some of the more well-known cases, four children died. All of these cases were linked to a well-known chain of fast-food restaurants. Several months later, five people in Oregon were hospitalized after eating meat tainted with E. coli bacteria. In the largest recall on record, federal investigators recently recalled 25 million pounds of hamburger meat produced by an Arkansas meat processor due to outbreaks of E. coli poisoning linked to the plant.[109] Currently, **the Centers for Disease Control estimates that there are over 20,000 cases of E. coli poisoning each year, resulting in 500 deaths. Some 70 percent of those cases can be linked directly to the consumption of hamburger meat.**[110]

Once the bacteria enters the body, it begins damaging the intestinal lining as well as the kidneys. Usually this results in bloody diarrhea. E. coli resides in the intestines and, therefore, in the feces of animals. During the slaughtering process, meat is likely to become contaminated by this deadly bacteria. Many question why, when the slaughtering procedure has changed little over the past few decades, E. coli has suddenly become such a great threat. In her monumental book *The Coming Plague*, health and science writer Laurie Garrett demonstrates that the unregulated use of large quantities of antibiotics in the raising of livestock has resulted in a more powerful "mutant strain" of the bacteria.

When one understands the operations of a modern slaughterhouse, such outbreaks of bacterial poisoning are really not surprising. Consider the following passage from Liane Cloresene-Casten's expose on the beef industry, which originally appeared in *Mother Jones* magazine. In a slaughterhouse she observed: "The headless carcasses wind around the killing floor at a rate of 325 per hour, where they are opened and the offal and paunch are removed. Immediately, 50 to 60 percent of the carcass becomes contaminated with fecal matter, urine from the leaking or breaking bladder, ingesta from the paunch, and bile from the liver. Once the spillage from the large intestine occurs, everything on the table including the by-products,becomes contaminated."[111]

To reduce the risk of E. coli poisoning, consumers are told to enjoy their meat well cooked. Ironically, though, the longer meat is cooked, the more it develops heterocyclic amines, a cancer-causing agent that forms when animal protein is heated excessively. In fact, **according to a recent National Cancer Institute study, those who eat their meat medium well-done to well-done are three times more likely to develop stomach cancer than those who eat meat rare.** Meat that is "charred," as often occurs in barbecuing, develops another class of carcinogens known as polycyclic aromatic hydrocarbons.[112]

The Bovine AIDS Problem

This may begin to sound like a sci-fi film at this point, but in fact the American beef and dairy herds have been found to have both a virus similar to human AIDS, known as bovine immunodeficiency virus (BIV), and bovine leukemia. On an average, the American herds have been shown to be infected by these diseases by about 20 percent and 80 percent respectively.[113]

Dioxin Contamination

Dioxin, a known human carcinogen that is a product of chlorine bleaching of paper, trash incineration, and burning of fossil fuels, is pervasive in the environment, and has been detected in foods. A study conducted in 1994 found that in foods purchased in an upstate New York supermarket, dioxin was detected in ground beef at a level of 1.5 ppt.[114] This exceeds the current EPA standard. For a further discussion of the hazards of exposure to dioxin, please see Chapter 5.

CHICKEN

As the health risks associated with red meat have become better known and its consumption continues to decline, many people have turned to poultry as a lower-fat alternative. Granted, poultry usually contains a bit less fat than red meat, but it is still saturated fat. Furthermore, as with meat, there are certain other risks associated with eating chicken. The biggest concern is over bacterial contamination, a problem that has become quite serious. According to the Center for Disease Control, each year nearly 2,000 Americans die from such bacterial poisoning.[115] Worse, however, the U.S. Department of Agriculture (USDA) reports that as many as 7 million Americans become infected annually from contaminated food.[116] The most common forms of bacteria include Salmonella and Campylobacter, and the latest estimates are that between 60 and 80 percent of chickens in the United States are

Nitrofurans, which may also be linked to an increased risk of cancer, are other contaminants found in chicken.

contaminated with these and other microorganisms, and a good number of these strains are now resistant to antibiotics.[117]

Much has been written about the unsanitary conditions in which animals are processed and how these conditions increase the chances of contamination. While the USDA, under fire by consumer advocates for failing to provide better monitoring and inspection, insists it has cracked down on chicken processors, a recent random sampling of chickens from supermarkets across the country suggests that considerable risk still exists. In this sampling, 30 different chickens were tested, including national brands, non-brands, kosher, and "free-range" varieties; 21 of the chickens were contaminated with Campylobacter, 12 with Listeria, and 8 with Salmonella.

Unwelcome Additives

In Chapter 5, we will look further at the toxicity of dioxin and some of the sources exposing us to this toxic chemical. Chicken is just one more source. Dioxin was declared a Class 1 carcinogen, or "known human carcinogen," by the International Agency for Research on Cancer (IARC), an arm of the World Health Organization, in February 1997. Currently, the U.S. FDA allows a one-part-per-trillion standard of dioxin in chicken.[118]

Nitrofurans, which may also be linked to an increased risk of cancer, are other contaminants found in chicken. They are intentionally added to chicken feed as a means of increasing growth rate. Gentian violet is a known human carcinogen which is intentionally added to chicken feed as a means of preventing fungal diseases, and preventing mold from developing on the feed.

The Cholesterol Is the Same, No Matter How You Slice It

Finally, since one of the primary motivating factors for many to switch from beef to chicken is the interest in lowering cholesterol levels, it should be noted that there is no difference between 4 ounces of beef and 4 ounces of chicken in terms of cholesterol content. Each serves up 100 mgs of cholesterol no matter how you cook it. So, though the intentions may be good, the switch from beef to chicken is nothing but a change in the color of the meat one is eating.

FISH

Fish has also become popular in recent years as a replacement for meat. Yet many of the popular fish, such as salmon and swordfish, are similar in fat content to poultry and meat. For instance, 52 percent of the calories in salmon come from fat. Like the meat it often replaces, fish also contains plenty of cholesterol.

Another increasing problem with fish is their level of contamination. Currently, 47 states have fish consumption advisories because of elevated levels of toxic chemicals found in certain species. PCBs, DDT, dioxin, and mercury are commonly found in ocean fish. In fact, fish are one of the most concentrated sources of PCBs today.* **Fish caught in U.S. rivers and lakes, with increasing frequency are found to contain benzene, hexachloride, chlordane, dieldrin, lindane, and toxaphene, all known carcinogens and some with endocrine disrupting potential.**[119]

Current estimates from the Center for Disease Control are that each year there are over 325,000 cases of illness caused by contaminated seafood. Unfortunately, many of the world's oceans, rivers, lakes, and streams have become great big rugs, under which tremendous amounts of toxic industrial waste are being swept. While we cannot easily see this waste, its presence is reflected in the increasing levels of contamination of fish.

Certain populations who depend on fish, including South American coastal villages and the Arctic Inuits, have been found to have exceptionally high concentrations of these contaminants in their bodies. It is well known that PCBs interfere with hormone activity and reproduction, as well as suppress immune system function.[120]

Consumption of some cold-water fish has been promoted on the grounds that they contain Omega-3 fatty acids, which are thought to provide protection against heart disease because they help prevent blood clotting. The popular press has failed to point out that vegetables such as spinach and broccoli, as well as some legumes, soybeans, tofu, dark leafy greens, pumpkin seeds, and particularly flaxseeds and flaxseed oil also are rich sources of the Omega-3s. However, taking fish oil capsules is more of the "magic bullet" thinking I presented earlier. No amount of fish oils is going to protect one from a hazardous diet and other risky lifestyle factors.

Some fish are carnivorous and thus high on the food chain. So when you eat them, you accumulate all the toxic chemicals from that fish in addition to the toxic chemicals it has bioaccumulated from all the fish it has eaten. Several fish varieties have been consistently found to have alarming levels of DDT, PCBs, and mercury. These include pike, walleye, bass, shark, and swordfish.[121]

As the hazards of open-water fish have become more well known, many consumers have turned to farmed fish. Fish farming (aquaculture) offers a whole host of other problems. Eric Hallerman of the Department of Fisheries and Wildlife Sciences at Virginia Polytechnic Institute, points out that fish farm conditions are so crowded that there are frequent outbreaks of disease, necessitating the use (and abuse) of antibiotics. Drug-resistant

---

*Please see Chapter 6 for a detailed look at the hazards of exposure to PCBs.

strains of bacteria are identified in these fish with increasing frequency. Some laboratory research has demonstrated that drug-resistance in fish pathogens can be transferred to human pathogens. [122]

PROBLEMS WITH MEAT, CHICKEN, AND FISH

- Pesticide residues (cancer promoter)
- Bacterial contamination (related to illnesses and death)
- Antibiotic residues (related to allergy and death)
- Low in vitamins and minerals (cancer protector)
- Void of phytochemicals (cancer protector)
- Void of fiber (cancer protector)
- Dioxin contamination (carcinogen)
- Industrial chemical contamination (carcinogen)
- High in cholesterol (heart disease promoter)
- High in saturated fat (cancer promoter, heart disease promoter)

IRRADIATED FOODS

Until actress Meryl Streep brought the pesticide Alar to the consciousness of America in 1987, few people had considered the possibility that our food contains residues of health-threatening chemicals. Since the Alar scare, not only have consumers become more aware of the potential risks of pesticide residues on our food, but the demand for organically grown fruits and vegetables (foods grown without synthetic pesticides and chemical fertilizers) has soared. The increase in the availability of organic foods has renewed a sense of food safety for many consumers who choose to buy them. To most of us, the thought that chemicals, some of which are known carcinogens, are being applied to many fruits, vegetables, grains, herbs, and spices, is haunting enough. Unfortunately, there is a new player in the world of food processing, one which, like many of the harmful pesticides currently used, may not be welcome at your dinner table. It's called food irradiation.

Food irradiation was developed in the 1950s by the Atomic Energy Commission when positive uses were being sought for the by-products of nuclear weapons production. The process involves exposing foods to either radioactive cobalt-60, a component of a nuclear reactor core, or cesium-137, a waste product of atomic bombs. **Irradiated foods may be exposed to as much as 300,000 rads (Radiation Absorbed Dose), the equivalent of 300,000 chest X-rays.**

Food irradiation has been shown to kill bacteria, tiny insects, and unseen parasites in meat, poultry, and fish that pose a risk of food poisoning. It also extends shelf life of foods.

Those in the business of food irradiation assert that it is the best way to eliminate the risk of food poisoning. Others point out that most poisonings are the result of poor cooking and processing of foods — problems that can be solved without resorting to food irradiation.

Food irradiation does have its hazards. For example, **irradiating food destroys beta carotene, up to one-third of the vitamin C content, and as much as 70 percent of vitamins A, B_1, and B_2.** It may also result in the formation of new chemicals called radiolytic products, including formaldehyde, peroxides, and benzene, all suspected human carcinogens, as well as

Irradiated foods may be exposed to as much as 300,000 rads (Radiation Absorbed Dose), the equivalent of 300,000 chest X-rays.

other unknown products. In testimony before the U.S. Congress, Dr. George L. Tritsch, a cancer researcher at Roswell Park Memorial Institute in New York, cautioned that consuming irradiated foods containing these radiolytic products could result in polyploidy, a condition involving cellular mutations.

According to Dr. Gary Gibbs, an irradiation authority and author of *The Food That Would Last Forever*, the Food and Drug Administration confirms that few studies have been conducted that support the long-term safety of irradiating foods for human consumption. Those that have been conducted have largely involved unwitting volunteers and have been poorly controlled. Further, the results of studies conducted on animals have not been encouraging. **Consider three University of Illinois studies in which mice were fed irradiated chicken, pork, milk, and carrots. In one study, 17 percent of the mice died from ruptured hearts. Others suffered burst blood vessels or testicular tumors.**[123]

Another area of concern that is largely ignored is the fact that a proliferation of food irradiating facilities necessarily means an increase in the production, transport, and accumulation of radioactive wastes.

Today, over 15 states, including Florida, California, and Colorado, have facilities licensed by the Nuclear Regulatory Commission (formerly the Atomic Energy Commission) to irradiate food. So far, the FDA has approved the irradiation of all fresh fruits, vegetables, pork, poultry, nuts, teas, and spices. One of the most commonly irradiated items in supermarkets are spices.

It is interesting to note that while proponents of irradiation claim studies have shown it safe, the Food and Drug Administration itself admits that when reviewed individually the studies are inadequate.[124]

Although foods that have been radiated are required to bare the radura (flowerlike) symbol and a warning label, if any of these foods are used as ingredients in prepared dishes, the manufacturer is not required to label the food accordingly. Furthermore, current law does not require restaurants to inform customers if dishes are prepared with irradiated foods.

Grocery retailers in general see food irradiation as a boon to business primarily because it will cut down on spoilage, which in turn means higher profits. Further, with the increasing number of food poisonings in the U.S., consumers are demanding greater assurance of food safety. You may want to ask the manager of your local market what their policy is regarding irradiated foods. Some markets, including Whole Foods and Wild Oats, have disclosed their policy not to carry any irradiated foods at all. Even more sweeping are the decisions of some states (New York and New Jersey) to outright ban the sale of irradiated foods within their borders.

FOODS THAT ARE FDA AND USDA APPROVED FOR IRRADIATION

1963: Wheat flour
1985: Pork
1986: Vegetables, spices
1992: Poultry
1997: Red meat

FATS AND OILS

Vegetable Oils

Contrary to the way they may appear in their shiny bottle when you bring them home, most all of the commercially available oils on the market today are rancid and a threat to your health. They are highly refined and subjected to a number of processes, including extraction using toxic solvents such as hexane (residues of which stay in the oil), and procedures such as defoaming, deodorizing, and degumming, as well as heating to extremely high temperatures. These processes destroy the vital nutrients such as phytosterols, beta carotene, chlorophyl, and vitamin E, and produce dangerous products such as free radicals. Oils in general are vulnerable to heat, oxygen, and light, and with exposure to these elements, degenerate further into unhealthy products. Finally, most oils contain dangerous pesticide residues, especially cottonseed oil because cotton is one of the most heavily sprayed crops. The exception are organically produced oils.

The best source of fats in the diet are those derived from whole foods such as whole grains, vegetables, legumes, and, in limited amounts, raw nuts and seeds. If oil is to be used, the most healthful would be expeller-pressed, extra virgin, organic olive oil, and then only in very small amounts. While research has consistently shown the highly monounsaturated fat of olive oil to be of significantly less risk than the polyunsaturated fat in safflower and corn oils,[125] this is not a license to indulge. Too much of any dietary fat is risky. A good alternative to cooking with oil is to either steam foods or sauté them with water or vegetable stock.

Margarine and Trans-Fats

Using margarine in place of butter has become very popular in recent years. However, margarine (and butter to a lesser degree) contains trans-fatty acids (TFAs). Recent studies have confirmed that TFAs are particularly unhealthy.[126] Convinced of the serious hazards associated with TFA consumption, the Netherlands has banned the sale of margarine containing trans-fats.

TFAs are created when food processors hydrogenate vegetable oils, a process that converts a liquid to a semisolid state. The process of hydrogenation involves adding hydrogen to the double bonds between carbon atoms in fatty acids, resulting in an otherwise liquid fat (oil) becoming semisolid. Hydrogenated fats are a food processor's dream, because the procedure makes the fat more durable, allowing a longer shelf life for products.

TRANS-FATTY ACID COMPOSITION OF SELECTED FOODS	
Margarine (stick)	up to 48%
(tub)	up to 44%
Candy bars	up to 39%
Vegetable shortening	up to 37%
French fries	up to 37%
Commercially baked goods	up to 34%
Butter	up to 15%

Here's where the problems begin. The process of hydrogenation makes an unsaturated fat into a saturated fat, the type of fat we know can elevate cholesterol levels and, as previously mentioned, promote certain cancers. Trans-fats also lower HDL ("good") cholesterol levels. Probably the most insidious result of hydrogenation is that it alters fat molecules from their natural "cis" (curved) configuration to an unnatural "trans" (jointed) configuration, which the body may have difficulty utilizing.[127] Ultimately, this molecular deformation may be carcinogenic.[128]

A study in the British medical journal *The Lancet*, which involved over 90,000 women, found that **those who consumed the most trans-fat-containing foods had a 50 percent higher risk of developing heart disease than those who consumed the least trans-fats.**[129] Other studies have shown that cancer deaths are higher among persons who consume the most trans-fats. **Eating trans-fats has also been directly linked to breast cancer.**[130]

You won't see "trans-fats" listed on the ingredient label of foods you buy, but you will see "hydrogenated" or "partially hydrogenated oil." Also, avoid foods that contain vegetable shortening and any foods that are deep-fried.

Olestra and Other "Non-Fat Fat"

Despite serious concern expressed by the Center for Science in the Public Interest (CSPI), the Food and Drug Administration (FDA) has recently approved the so-called "fake fat" called Olestra, manufactured by Procter & Gamble. The synthetic fat is a sucrose polyester synthesized from sugar and vegetable oil.

Unlike Simplesse, another artificial fat (made from milk and egg white protein) that was approved by the FDA in 1990, Olestra is heat stable and can therefore be used in baking and frying. Because of its chemical structure, Olestra molecules are too large for the body to absorb and therefore are non-caloric. However, some potential problems have been identified with the fake fat. CSPI maintains that the synthetic fat binds with important vitamins, including A, D, and E, as well as some carotenoids, including beta carotene, and prevents the body from absorbing and utilizing them. Vitamins A and E and certain carotenoids are believed to be important antioxidants that help protect cells from free-radical damage, thereby reducing the risk of certain cancers, coronary heart disease, and cataracts. CSPI also reports the fat may cause gastrointestinal problems such as bloating, nausea, and diarrhea.

The recent approval allows Olestra to be used only in snack foods such as potato chips and crackers. Other fat substitutes that you may see on labels soon include Caprenin (Proctor & Gamble), Trailblazer (Kraft General Foods), and Simplese (Monsanto).

As studies have shown, all of the foods mentioned in this chapter may pose various risks to your health, particularly when they make up a large part of the diet. By eliminating these foods from your diet, you may sharply reduce your chance of developing not only breast cancer but a host of other chronic degenerative diseases. Yet diet is just one part of a synergistic preventive equation. To maximize risk reduction one must apply each of the seven steps discussed herein. In Part Two we will discuss specific steps you can take to reduce your risk, such as changing your diet to include more healthful alternatives, reducing exposure to hazardous chemicals, and applying other simple lifestyle changes.

CHAPTER SIX

The Chemical Connection

Earth is awash in a sea of toxic chemicals. They are found in increasing concentration in our food, soil, water, air—even in the raindrops that fall upon the planet. The average human now carries in his or her body the residues of some two-hundred synthetic chemicals that did not exist at the turn of the twentieth century. An increasing number of studies suggest that our ever-increasing exposure to these chemicals may be playing a role in a variety of health problems humans face, not the least of

Researchers have found breast cancer rates to be 6.5 times higher in counties with toxic waste dumps than in counties without.

which being the epidemic of breast cancer.[162] In fact, today there are over four-hundred studies in the medical literature demonstrating that a variety of chemicals cause breast cancer in animals.

Chemicals can raise our risk in a variety of ways. Some are known or suspected carcinogens, while others are cancer promoters. Many chemicals wreak havoc on the body's hormone economy, and may thereby heighten risk of hormone-dependent cancers such as breast and prostate cancer. A large number of chemicals can cause damage to the immune system, rendering us more susceptible to cancer.

The degree to which each of us is exposed on a daily basis is difficult to grasp. In this chapter, I am going to give you a perspective on the chemical problem and how it may be contributing to the rising incidence of cancer. Then, in Chapter 12, you will learn how best to minimize your exposure.

According to the Environmental Protection Agency's Toxic Release Inventory, last year we dispersed some five-hundred billion pounds of toxic chemicals into the environment, 4 billion pounds of which were pesticides. There are currently over 80,000 chemicals in regular use, with one-thousand to two-thousand new chemicals added to the list each year.[131] Current estimates are that a mere 3 percent have been tested for carcinogenicity.

While some chemicals are used directly in the production of food (insecticides, herbicides, and fungicides) and may thereby pose a risk via diet, others are used to fumigate homes and commercial structures. Still others are used by municipalities to control the growth of plants along highways and city streets. Some chemicals are ingredients in common household cleaners, bug killers, spot removers, and even personal cosmetics. Even the process of dry-cleaning clothes exposes us to toxic chemicals. A large amount of these chemicals end up in our waterways (rivers, lakes, streams) and, ultimately, our oceans.

Other sources of chemicals in the environment include toxic waste dumps (of which the Environmental Protection Agency now lists over 32,000) and illegal hazardous chemical dump sites—an indeterminable number. It is noteworthy that researchers have found breast cancer rates to be 600 percent higher in counties with toxic waste dumps than in counties without. In general, the closer women live to such dumps, the higher the death rate from breast cancer.*

Another source of toxic chemicals can be found in your own home. Do you have pets? An EPA study suggests that about 50 percent of U.S. households do. Chances are that you treat your dog or cat with a variety of flea powders and sprays which are toxic not only to the fleas but to pets and humans as well.

Millions of American women either have their hair professionally colored or apply do-it-yourself dyes at home each month. According to numerous studies, something as seemingly benign as hair coloring exposes women to numerous chemicals that appear to elevate risk of breast cancer.[132] Fortunately, there are safer alternatives. (See Resources).

---

*Najem, G.R., et al., *Preventive Medicine* 14 (1985):620-35; Griffith, Jack, et al., *Archives of Environmental Health* 44 (1989):69-74; Najem, G.R., et al., *International Journal of Epidemiology* 14 (1985):528-37.

Many American households and apartment complexes now rely on lawn care services that apply toxic chemicals to lawns year round. One in five Americans applies such chemicals themselves. Whether absorbed through skin or inhaled during application, or brought into the family home on shoes or the feet of a pet, these chemicals pose a serious risk.

Endocrine-Disrupting Chemicals

Endocrine-disruptor, estrogen mimic, and xenoestrogen are some of the names used to describe industrial and agricultural chemicals that when ingested can disrupt normal hormone function and apparently wreak havoc on both human and animal health. Examples of chemicals that have been identified as endocrine disruptors include polychlorinated biphenyls (PCBs), dioxins, and some pesticides, including the notorious DDT.

Recently, experts in the fields of endocrinology, immunology, pathology, biology, and anthropology have begun working together to understand how these chemicals may be playing a role in the dramatic rise in cases of breast, prostate and testicular cancer, undescended testicles, lowered sperm count, and immune deficiency disorders worldwide.

To understand how these chemicals can affect our health, it is essential to have a basic understanding of the endocrine system. The system is composed of a variety of hormones, including estrogen, testosterone, adrenaline, and insulin, and the glands that secrete them, including the ovaries, testicles, pituitary, adrenals, thyroid, and pancreas.

Hormones can be thought of as chemical messengers that are responsible for initiating and/or supporting a myriad number of processes in the body. These include sexual development, brain development, pregnancy, and metabolism. When hormones are transported to and bind with target cells, this can initiate a process. Hormones activate processes at astonishingly minuscule doses. To convey their potency, Theo Colborn, Ph.D., senior scientist at the World Wildlife Fund, asks us to "imagine a quantity so infinitesimally small by thinking of a drop of gin in a train of tank cars full of tonic. One drop in 660 tank cars would be one part in a trillion; such a train would be six miles long."

---

*Gurunathan, Somia, et al., *Environmental Health Perspectives* 106 (1998):9-16; **103 (1995):582-587.

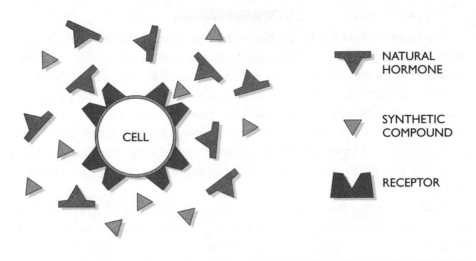

NATURAL HORMONE

SYNTHETIC COMPOUND

RECEPTOR

CELL

Reprinted with permission of World Wildlife Fund, Canada.

The Lock and Key System

In order for hormones to exert their effect, they must first be delivered to special receptor proteins found on cells. Think of the hormone as the key and the receptor as the lock. Hormones and receptors are highly specialized, and only with the correct fit can the lock be opened and a process initiated. However, endocrine-disrupting chemicals manage to deceive the receptors (see illustration). In doing so, they can effectively unlock the cell and expose its DNA, and thereby initiate a process such as cell proliferation, or they can simply block the receptor site so that natural hormones are unable to be received and activate a process. Some of these chemicals can "super-activate" a process, resulting in a much stronger effect than natural hormones would illicit.

Endocrine-disrupting chemicals can also interfere with the natural production of hormones in the body, both androgens (male hormones) and estrogens (female hormones). Additionally, while natural hormones are metabolized and excreted from the body after use, some chemicals can interfere with enzymes that assist in the natural process of eliminating hormones from the body. By stifling this process, higher than intended levels of hormones are available to receptors. Finally, unlike natural hormones, xenoestrogens can remain in the body for decades, keeping hormone levels artificially elevated.*

---

*For a detailed examination of the effects of endocrine-disrupting chemicals on both wildlife and humans, please see *Our Stolen Future: Are We Threatening Our Fertility, Intelligence, and Survival?—A Scientific Detective Story* (New York: Dutton, 1996).

The Wildlife Warning

The same sorts of health problems we are seeing in humans today were showing up in wildlife decades ago. In fact, it was the increasing incidence of deformities and other health problems occurring in animals that led scientists to begin looking at the role certain chemicals could be playing in human developmental problems and disease later in life. Since the endocrine systems of animals and humans function in the same fashion and with hormones that are chemically alike, it makes sense that health effects occurring in animals as a result of chemical exposure may well be a concern for humans.

With increasing frequency, scientists are finding thyroid dysfunction in birds and fish, scaleless fish with facial tumors, birth defects such as deformed genitalia and hermaphroditism, infertility in fish, birds, and mammals, metabolic abnormalities, demasculinization, and suppressed immune function.

Today, about 50 percent of green sea turtles are now found with huge facial tumors called fibropapillomas.* In 1988 there was the sudden death of 25,000 seals in the Baltic Sea. A year later, over 1,000 dolphins washed up dead. In both cases, autopsies revealed high concentrations of endocrine-disrupting chemicals in the animals' flesh. Scientists believe the chemical exposure lead to compromised function of the immune system, leaving the creatures vulnerable to diseases to which they would normally have been impervious.

More recently, British researchers from Brunel University suspect that endocrine-disrupting chemicals are causing the feminization of large numbers of fish. After discovering male fish born with ovaries and eggs instead of sperm ducts, they began researching the levels of endocrine-disrupting chemicals in eight rivers throughout Great Britain. Most of the sites they used to study the fish and measure chemical contamination are downstream of treatment plants. In two of the eight study sites, 100 percent of the male fish sampled had feminized reproductive tracts. In the other six sites, the rate of feminization ranged from 20 percent to 80 percent.

In Florida, panthers are showing serious health problems, including sterility, lowered sperm count, suppressed immune function, and dysfunction of the thyroid gland. In one case, over 70 percent of the male panthers examined suffered from cryptorchidism, in which the testicles do not descend from the abdomen. Testicle descention is signaled by the male

---

*Raloff, Janet, *Science News* 146 (1994):8-9.

hormone testosterone and occurs late in the gestation period. If the hormone signals are somehow blocked, the testicles may remain, like ovaries, in the abdomen. Cryptorchidism is appearing with increasing frequency not only in male animals but in human babies around the world.

The Mystery Unfolds

Until recently, most discoveries of a chemical's propensity to disrupt hormone activity were made quite by accident. One of the more well-known cases was reported in *Our Stolen Future*. At Tufts University, Ana Soto and Carlos Sonnenschein were studying the process by which cell multiplication goes awry—the central theme in cancer. Dr. Soto and her colleague were using estrogen-dependent human breast cells in their work. They already knew that if they added estrogen to their tissue samples, cell multiplication would occur. When they added an estrogen-free serum to the sample, they found cell multiplication would stop.

That material, a plasticizer called nonylphenol, as it turns out, mimics the activity of estrogen.

One day they discovered that even in the samples where estrogen-free serum was used, cell multiplication appeared to be occurring. Mystified by this occurrence, they set out on a search to determine what had caused this unexpected interference with their well-controlled experiment. With great cost, frustration, and lost time, they eventually learned that, in an effort to make its tubes less brittle, the manufacturer of the special lab tubes they were using had recently started using a new material in its manufacturing process. The university was unaware of the product change. That material, a plasticizer called nonylphenol, it turns out, mimics the activity of estrogen.

Today we know that nonylphenol, an estrogen mimic, is used not only in plastic lab tubes, but also in many other materials, such as polyvinyl chloride (PVC) and other common plastics. It is even used to synthesize a component found in contraceptive creams. What is worse, each year in the United States we manufacture some 400 million pounds of industrial detergents, pesticides, and even personal care products that contain alkylphenol polyethoxylates, which, when acted upon by bacteria occurring in our body, the environment, and sewage treatment plants, can release nonylphenol.

EDCs, Food Packaging, and Water Containers

Another estrogen mimic has been identified called bisphenol-A (BPA). An additive in polycarbonate plastics, it is a common ingredient in the large blue plastic jugs that are used to transport and store "purified water," canned food linings, and even dental sealant and fillings. In one study, significant quantities of bisphenol-A were found in half of 20 brands of canned food tested.[134]

Alkylphenols and another plastisizer called phthalates are commonly used in the manufacture of children's toys, cellular phones, and the abundance of plastic adorning the interior of newer cars. Phthalates are also found in plastic food wrap and "to-go" paper food containers. Styrene cups, plates and eating utensils are particularly problematic because when hot foods or liquids come in contact with them, endocrine-disrupting chemicals and other carcinogenic chemicals may migrate into the food.* Both phthalates and alkylphenols are not only endocrine-disruptors, but are classified as probable carcinogens.

The Power of Synergy

Most of the research to date has focused on the ability of a single chemical to interfere with endocrine activity. The reality, however, is that humans and animals are rarely exposed to a single agent. Instead, the chemical contamination commonly found in drinking water, foodstuff, and even personal care products, is often a cocktail of different compounds. As an example, some pesticides have been identified as endocrine disruptors. As will be seen in Chapter 10, some tests of fruit have revealed up to eight different pesticide residues on a single apple, some known endocrine disruptors. Fish caught in the Great Lakes region typically are contaminated with a variety of known endocrine disruptors. What are the effects of such combination exposures? At this time, we are not certain, but preliminary research suggests that such contamination may pose a far more potent risk than individual agents.[135]

In October 1998, after a congressional mandate, the Environmental Protection Agency (EPA) announced plans to begin screening chemicals to determine if they are endocrine disruptors. While the initial plan targets 15,000 chemicals, the goal is to eventually test all of the 80,000 chemicals in use. While EPA assistant administrator Lynn Goldman called the task a "technological challenge," the magnitude of what must ultimately be done

---

*Jobling, S., et al., *Environmental Health Perspectives* 103 (1995):582-87.

is difficult to grasp. Many questions remain about how the test will be implemented. For instance, what doses, combinations, and in what priority should the chemicals be tested?

Peter Montague, Ph.D., director of the Environmental Research Foundation, reveals that the enormity of the task surpasses our financial and person-power capacities. He cautions: "To test just the commonest 1,000 toxic chemicals in unique combinations of 3 would require at least 166 million different experiments (and this disregards the need to study varying doses given to animals at varying times during their lives). If we wanted to conduct the 166 million experiments in just 20 years, we would have to complete 8.3 million tests each year. The U.S. presently has the capacity to conduct only a few hundred such tests each year. Just training sufficient personnel to conduct 8.3 million animal tests each year is beyond our national capacity."

OTHER CHEMICAL CONCERNS

Dioxin

Dioxin is actually a collective term for a family of 75 chemicals. It is a by-product created in the making of chlorine-bleached paper, paper towels, paper plates and cups, napkins, facial tissues, tampons, toilet paper, diapers, and tea bags, as well as in the process of burning plastic-containing trash and burning fossils fuels. In fact, ironically, medical waste incineration is the second largest source of dioxin in the U.S. today. The reason is that a large part of medical waste (IV bags, gloves etc.) is PVC products which are composed of about 50 percent chlorine.

Dioxin is a known endocrine-disruptor (it both mimics female hormones and blocks male hormones), carcinogen, and immune system suppresser, which also disrupts the central nervous system and the reproductive system, and interferes with normal growth and development.[136]

A recent study revealed that humans now carry enough dioxin in their bodies to create a cancer risk hundreds of times as large as the "acceptable" cancer risk defined by the Environmental Protection Agency.[137] **While the EPA has established an _acceptable_ exposure level for dioxin, it confirms that there is _no safe_ level of exposure.**

Some researchers believe that dioxin, even at extremely small doses, can reduce the number of T and B cells in the immune system, and that in the unborn child, it may prevent the immune system from developing properly, potentially sentencing the child to a lifetime of compromised immune function.

Studies have shown that chronic exposure to dioxin can cause endometriosis (disease of the uterine lining) in monkeys.[138] Some 9 million American women suffer from endometriosis. Tests consistently show the presence of dioxin in human breast milk.[139] Because the dioxin produced in the above stated industries eventually makes its way into the food chain where it bioaccumulates, dioxin is also a common contaminant of meat, poultry, and fish. **In fact, the EPA maintains that 95 percent of human exposure to dioxins occurs chiefly through eating red meat, fish, and dairy products.**[140]

Polychlorinated Biphenyls (PCBs)

PCBs encompass a family of 209 different synthetic organochlorine compounds designated as carcinogens by the U.S. Department of Health and Human Services and the International Agency for Research on Cancer. PCBs are also endocrine-disruptors, and have been linked to immune system damage and reproductive and growth disturbances.

Because of their insulative and nonflammable properties, PCBs were at one time commonly used as coolants and lubricants in electrical transformers, as coating in carbonless paper, in caulking, synthetic resins, waxes, asphalt, rubbers, paints, and in the manufacture of pesticides. From 1929 to 1977, over 1 million tons of PCBs were manufactured, 370,000 tons of which have already been released into the environment.

Today, even in the absence of PCB production, human exposure continues by way of antiquated electrical appliances, transformers, and even old fluorescent lighting fixtures, televisions, and refrigerators—any such equipment that was manufactured prior to 1977. As older equipment heats up, PCBs can leak out and vaporize into the air. Enormous quantities of PCBs have been introduced into the environment through a variety of means, including incineration, vaporization of paints and coatings, through equipment leaks and uncontained landfills (PCBs have been detected in over two-hundred waste sites), and of course, through intentional dumping of waste into the ocean.

PCBs are fat-soluble and therefore concentrate in the fat of animals and humans. A prime place for concentration is in breast tissue. Consider that after only six months of breast feeding, a baby born in the U.S. today will have received five times the "allowable" daily intake of PCBs.[141] In adults, PCB exposure is most likely to occur through the consumption of fatty foods such as meats, cheese, and butter. Fish and shellfish are considered prime sources of PCB contamination. According to the Agency for Toxic Substances and Disease Registry (ATSDR), some of the highest concentrations of PCBs are found among people who eat more than six pounds (twelve meals) of fish a year.

Polyvinyl Chloride (PVC)

Polyvinyl chloride is pervasive in our world today. It is used to manufacture garden hoses, children's toys, outdoor furniture, and credit cards, as well as numerous other items. In the medical world, PVC is often used in IV bags, ventilator tubing, examination gloves, patient ID-bracelets, mattress covers, and oral airways.

Vinyl chloride, which is used to make PVC, is a known human carcinogen that has been linked to increased risk of breast cancer in several studies.[142] One study showed that for women who breathed vinyl chloride vapors in the workplace, there was a 36 percent increase is breast cancer mortality.*

Many items constructed of PVC also contain the toxic plastisizer known as phthalates (pronounced thalates). The most common pthalates used are di-ethylhexyl-phthalate (DEHP), di-isodecylphthalate (DIDP), and di-isononyl-phthalate. As indicated earlier, phthalates are not only endocrine-disruptors, they have been linked with cancer (in animals and humans), kidney and liver damage, and lowered sperm counts in rats, as well as damage to the reproductive organs. Since phthalates are not chemically bound to PVC they have a tendency to leach out of plastic, and may end up in foods or even children's mouths after contact with plastic toys.

PVC use doubled in the U.S. between 1980 and 1995. Ironically, a good deal of PVC use is justified on the basis that it is a plastic and therefore recyclable. In truth, however, PVC is the least recyclable of all plastics in use today. The reason is that PVC is composed of so many additional chemicals that the process of recycling it is simply too costly. The EPA estimates that less than 0.5 percent of all post-consumer PVC is recovered annually.[143]

Perchloroethylene and the Dangers of Dry Cleaning

Could something as seemingly benign as dry cleaning be playing a role in the escalating rates of cancer? Recent research suggests so. Contrary to the term, there is nothing dry about dry cleaning. The process involves using heavy-duty industrial solvents, the most common being per-chloroethylene (called perc), a petroleum-derived hydrocarbon with attached chlorine molecules. Each year, the 35,000 dry-cleaning establish ments in the U.S. and Canada use some 300 million pounds of this chemical. About 287 pounds of this is released into the environment (air, water, and soil) daily.[144]

In the U.S., perc has been detected in seafood, beef, cow's milk, rainwater, tap water, and even human breast milk. Perc outgassing from dry-cleaned clothes can be measured in home air after garments are hung in the closet.[145] A major concern is over perc being absorbed through the skin when a person wearing dry-cleaned garments perspires.

Unfortunately, even if you don't have your clothes dry-cleaned, you may still be exposed to perc through food, water and air. Simply living or working above a dry-cleaning business can be risky. A survey found that over 80 percent of apartments located above dry cleaners contained ambient levels of perc that exceeded state guidelines.*

The good news is that there are alternatives to dry cleaners rapidly opening across the nation. Called "wet cleaners," these businesses offer garment cleaning without the use of perc or any other toxic chemical.

WHAT'S IN THE WATER YOU'RE DRINKING?

Our bodies have a great need for water, and in Chapter 11 we will explore this need in greater detail. Unfortunately, no longer can we turn on the kitchen faucet and assume we are getting safely treated water. The average municipal water source is loaded with toxic contaminants, including asbestos, lead, cadmium, and other heavy metals, nitrates, fluoride, pesticides, chlorine, and trihalomethanes,[146] antibiotics, hormones, tranquilizers, pain killers, and chemotherapy drugs used to treat cancer.**

According to the EPA, over 700 chemicals, including 98 different pesticides, had been identified in drinking water by 1984. Just between 1991 and 1992, federal agencies received reports of 34 outbreaks involving disease-tainted drinking water. Some 50 percent of those cases were the result of the malfunction of purification facilities. Probably the most well known and lethal case in recent years was the 1993 outbreak of cryptosporidium in Milwaukee. Over 400,000 people were sickened and 100 people died before the problem was brought under control. As previously mentioned, the chemical perchloroethylene (perc) is the industrial solvent used by 94 percent of America's dry cleaners today. Perc has been linked with leukemia and cancer of the pancreas, bladder, kidney, and cervix.[147] This chlorinated hydrocarbon has been detected in 34 percent of municipal water systems in

---

*Upstairs, Downstairs: Perchloroethylene in the Air in Apartments Above New York City Dry-Cleaners. (Consumers Union: New York, 1995); Clothed in Controversy: The Risk to New Yorkers from Dry-Cleaning Emissions and What Can Be Done About It. (Office of the Public Advocate for the City of New York, 1994).
**Raloff, Janet, *Science News* 153 (1998):187-189.

36 cities surveyed by the U.S. government.[148] If you live in California and drink unfiltered water, **you may be one of over a million citizens whose water contains a confirmed breast cancer-causing compound with the tongue-twisting name dibromochloropropane.**

The latest report from the Environmental Protection Agency (EPA) found the water systems of 819 cities providing service to 30 million people exceeded the "safe" lead levels established by the Safe Water Drinking Act.[149] The Centers for Disease Control and the EPA have warned that because of increasing outbreaks of cryptosporidium bacteria, cancer patients, organ transplant recipients, and anyone with a weakened immune system should avoid drinking tap water.

The sources of water contaminants are numerous. They include runoff of pesticides from agricultural areas (especially in the Midwest), commercial lawn fertilizers, leaks from improperly stored or dumped toxic waste, landfills, paints, septic tanks used in rural areas, and antiquated sewer systems that fail to properly treat water before releasing it into rivers and lakes. Heavy metals such as cadmium and lead often find their way into the water system from aging galvanized pipes. Nitrates, a known human carcinogen, are usually the result of chemical fertilizer runoff. Even hospitals have been found to dump low-level radioactive waste into the sewers.[150]

Fluoride

Too many health problems are associated with fluoride for us to sit back and hope that if we put it in our water, it will take care of our teeth. The fact is that the fluoride used in drinking water is a toxic by-product of the aluminum and fertilizer industries.[151] **Evidence shows fluoride toxicity to be "linked with genetic damage in plants and animals, birth defects in humans, especially Down's syndrome, plus a whole series of allergic reactions ranging from fatigue, headaches, urinary tract irritations, diarrhea, and many others."**[152]

For years we have accepted as dogma the notion that fluoride in our drinking water helps prevent tooth decay. No scientific research exists to support its use in drinking water. On the contrary, research in the 1950s suggested that fluoridated water did nothing to reduce the incidence of cavities. With some of the highest levels of drinking water fluoridation, the United States also has the distinction of having one of the highest levels of tooth decay. This should tell us something.

HAZARDS OF CHEMICALS THAT MAY BE IN YOUR WATER

CONTAMINANT	HEALTH EFFECT	SOURCE
ENDRIN	Toxic to nervous system and kidneys	Banned pesticide used on cotton, grains and orchards
LINDANE	Toxic to nervous system, kidneys, and possible carcinogen	Pesticide used on soil, foliage, and seeds
METHOXYCHLOR	Toxic to nervous system, kidneys	Pesticide used on fruits and vegetables
2, 4-D	Toxic to liver and kidneys	Herbicide used to control weeds in agriculture, forests, aquatic environments
2, 4, 5-TP SILVEX	Toxic to liver and kidneys	Herbicides. Banned
TOXAPHENE	Carcinogen	Pesticide used on corn, cotton and grains
BENZENE	Carcinogen	Gasoline tanks, solvents, pharmaceuticals, pesticides, plastics, and paints
PERCHLOROETHELENE	Carcinogen	Common dry-cleaning solvent
P-DICHLOROBENZENE	Likely carcinogen	Pesticides, moth balls, air deodorizers
1, 2-DICHLOROETHANE	Likely carcinogen	Pesticide manufacturing
1, 1-DICHLOROETHYLENE	Toxic to liver and kidneys	Manufacturing of plastics, dyes, perfumes, paints
VINYL CHLORIDE	Carcinogen	Polyvinyl chloride pipes (PVC), solvents, industrial waste from manufacture of plastics, and synthetic rubber
CHLORINE	Carcinogen	Intentionally introduced into most municipal water systems, swimming pools and hot tubs
HEAVY METALS	Toxic to nervous system, linked to Alzheimer's and Parkinson's disease, kidney, and brain damage.	Industrial waste
NITRATES	Carcinogen	Fertilizers
FLUORIDE	Linked with birth defects, urinary tract infections. Possible skin mouth and bone carcinogen[151]	Introduced into most municipal water systems intentionally

Source: "You and Your Water," *EPA Journal* 12 (7), September 1986.

In truth, tooth decay is primarily due to the large consumption of sugars in the United States, coupled with poor tooth maintenance (i.e., faulty and inconsistent brushing and flossing habits). Furthermore, in areas where the municipal water systems are high in fluoride, children may develop permanent rust-like stains or "mottling" on their teeth.

Four studies published in the *Journal of the American Medical Association* (JAMA) since 1990 have indicated that hip fracture rates are higher in communities where fluoridation is used in the municipal water system. Other research has linked fluoridation with damage to the central nervous system, genetic damage, [153] cancer, and lowered I.Q. in children. [154]

It is noteworthy that the National Federation of Federal Employees, a union comprised of scientists, engineers, lawyers, and other professionals at the headquarters of the Environmental Protection Agency, professionals who are charged with assessing the safety of drinking water, has chosen to sponsor the California state initiative to prohibit fluoridation of drinking water. In a formal statement made by Dr. J. William Hirzy, vice president of the NFFE, it was said, **"We conclude that the health and welfare of the public is not served by the addition of this substance . . . (fluoride) a hazardous waste of the fertilizer industry . . . to the public water supply."[155]** At least 14 countries have already come to the same conclusion and outlawed fluoridation of drinking water.

Chlorine

Chlorine is deliberately placed in our drinking water system as a means of "purifying" it. The reality is quite the contrary. While chlorine does kill bacteria and other potentially offending matter, dozens of studies have linked chlorination with liver, kidney, rectal, brain, stomach, and bladder cancers,[156] cancer of the breast, prostate, and testicles, and learning disabilities in children.[157] Dr. Sandra Steingraber, author of *Living Downstream*, addressed the chlorine problem succinctly when she said, "Giving people cancer in order to ensure them a water supply safe from disease-causing microbes is not necessary." Recently, a **U.S.-Canadian advisory commission established expressly to examine the health problems associated with chlorine released a statement urging that both countries place an immediate ban on the sale and production of chlorine because of what it called "startling health problems."[158]** It appears that this report fell upon deaf ears.

Chlorine is by far one of the most common toxic chemicals in use today, and its negative effects are enormous.

Chlorine has a tendency to interact negatively with other substances. Natural organic matter and other substances, when mixed with chlorine, create a chemical reaction that results in the production of cancer-causing trihalomethanes (THMs) such as chloroform, compounds that promote the production of harmful free radicals.[159]

The production of PVCs, which are used in the manufacture of furnishings, children's toys, auto parts, and even hospital supplies, as well as hundreds of other products, is the largest and fastest growing use of chlorine today. Yet chlorine enters our environment in many other forms, especially through swimming pools and hot tubs. I recently walked into the lobby of a motel in a small town in Illinois. I had simply wanted to check-in and get the key to my room. When I entered the lobby, I was overwhelmed by the smell of chlorine in the air. I felt an urgent need to get out of there as quickly as possible. After further investigation, I learned that the motel was built around a very large indoor swimming pool, which was obviously heavily treated with chlorine. The chlorine fumes entered the air and made their way into the nearby dining room and lobby, and it seemed that the employees, having become acclimated, were unaware of the hazard to which they were being exposed.

Chlorine is purposefully added to municipal water systems to control bacteria growth. For this, it does a wonderful job. However, once that job is done, it remains in the water and is consumed at the tap, posing a serious risk to our health and that of the environment.

Chlorine is also intentionally added to swimming pools, hot tubs, and Jacuzzis® to control bacteria. In facilities with heavy public use, such as health clubs and community pools, chlorine tends to be added in bountiful amounts. A preponderance of evidence indicates that swimming and soaking in chlorine-rich water is a highly hazardous activity that should be avoided at all cost.

Lead

Lead contamination from drinking water has become a big problem. The most recent EPA survey found 130 municipal water systems exceeding "safe" lead levels and 10 systems with levels that exceeded allowable levels by four times. Excess levels of lead are known to cause damage to the brain, nervous system, kidneys, and red blood cells. Lead has been found to be a particular threat to children and pregnant women, since even low levels have been found to cause anemia and damage to children's immune system, low birth weight (a leading cause of infant mortality), learning disabilities, behavioral problems, and retarded growth. Homes and apartment complexes constructed before the 1980s were likely to have had pipes installed that contained lead. After that time, lead regulations forced builders to use lead-free materials.

THE DANGERS OF PESTICIDES

Today there are some 20,000 different pesticides manufactured, with over 4 billion pounds used worldwide annually, 2 billion of which are used in the U.S. alone. Estimates are that, worldwide, 25 million people are poisoned by pesticides annually,* (nearly 50 people every minute). The potential health effects from pesticide exposure are varied and include acute poisoning, neurological and reproductive effects, brain damage, birth defects, infertility, suppression of the immune system, and cancer. Health costs associated with pesticide use in the U.S. are conservatively estimated to be $780 million a year.**

Consider that pesticides are habitually used in schools (see Chapter 18), parks, health clubs, airplanes, and restaurants, and on golf courses, roadsides, and athletic fields. According to the EPA, consumers spend some $1.2 billion annually to apply pesticides to their own homes and gardens.

According to the National Academy of Sciences, an astonishing 1 million cases of cancer may develop in this generation from pesticide exposure through foods alone.[160] When one considers just how pervasive pesticide use is in agriculture, such an estimate becomes less surprising. For example, consider the herbicide atrazine. This chemical, a known endocrine-disruptor, is used on 70 percent of cornfields in America. So far, atrazine has been linked with breast cancer in animals and ovarian cancer in women.*** In the Midwest, atrazine is a major contaminant of groundwater. Vinclozolin, a common fungicide associated with birth defects including genital deformities, is regularly detected on beans, peas, and onions.****

The Washington, D.C.-based Environmental Working Group examined FDA data for a three-year period and found startling pesticide contamination of foods. Over 80 percent of peach, apple, and celery samples contained residues of one or more pesticides, 12 of which are known carcinogens, 17 are confirmed neurotoxins, and 11 are endocrine-disruptors or interfere with reproduction.

---

*Matthiessen, C., "The Day the Poison Stopped Working," *Mother Jones*, March/April 1992.
**Solomon, Gina M., et al., Trouble on the Farm, Executive Summary, Natural Resources Defense Council, October 1998.
***Biradar, D.P., et al., *Archives of Environmental Contamination and Toxicology* 28 (1995):13-17; Donna, A., et al., *Carcinogenesis* 5 (1984):941-42.
****Gray, L.E., et al., *Toxicology and Applied Pharmacology* 129 (1994):46-52.

Data collected in the EPA's National Home and Garden Pesticide survey suggests that about 82 percent of American households currently use one or another form of pesticide in their home. One of the most common applications is by way of insecticide foggers. It was recently shown that such foggers pose a serious threat to household members long after their initial activation. In one study, the chemical ingredient chlorpyrifos, one of the most widely used ingredients in home foggers, was still accumulating on household furnishings, carpet, pillows, and, even more disconcerting, children's plastic toys, a full two weeks after application.*

No-Pest strips pose another serious risk. These insecticide strips contain a potent toxic chemical called DDVP. The chemical is released into the air and inhaled by all occupants of the home. DDVP is associated with an increased risk of all types of cancer and causes breast tumors in animals. According to a recent study in the *Journal of Pesticide Reform*, the EPA estimates that occupants of households with such pest strips have a cancer risk 10 times greater than professional pesticide applicators who use the same chemical.[133]

A study by the North Carolina Pesticide Board found that 27 percent of water wells they sampled were contaminated with 31 different pesticides, many of which are confirmed to cause cancer, birth defects, and genetic damage, or harm the endocrine and immune systems.[163]

In the 1980s, millions of Southern California residents were involuntarily "dusted" on a repeated basis with the endocrine-disrupting pesticide malathion. After sightings of the Mediterranean fruit fly, and fearing a crop infestation, officials concluded that nighttime aerial spraying of neighborhoods was in order.

While there is no conclusive evidence to date showing pesticides *cause* breast cancer, and a few that show no correlation, the preponderance of studies suggest a link.[161] In fact, the collective evidence is disconcerting. As mentioned in Chapter 4, a study conducted at Mt. Sinai Medical Center in New York found that malignant breast tissue samples contained up to 60 percent higher concentrations of pesticide residues when compared to healthy tissue. Another study conducted by Finnish researchers found that women with the highest levels of common pesticide residues in their breast tissue were ten times more likely to develop breast cancer than women with the lowest levels.[162]

---

*Gurunathan, Somia, et al., *Environmental Health Perspectives* 106 (1998):9-16.

DDT

The insecticide DDT is likely one of the most notorious chemicals humans have created. A confirmed endocrine-disruptor, DDT use in the U.S. was banned in 1972 because of concern over it being carcinogenic. However, hundreds of tons are still manufactured for use throughout the world, including Mexico, India, South America, and Africa, primarily as a means for controlling the spread of malaria. In reviewing U.S. Customs shipping records, the Foundation for Advancements in Science and Education (FASE) found that in one 12-month period, a staggering 300 tons of DDT was shipped from the U.S. to Peru.*

You won't ever have to travel to these parts of the world to be exposed to DDT. This is because the substance makes its way to even the most remote parts of the planet via air and ocean currents. More recently, with expanded agricultural imports, DDT is also coming back to America by way of exotic fruits, vegetables, and other foods grown in countries that still use the compound.

Despite the fact that DDT use was formally banned in the U.S. over 20 years ago, U.S. Fish and Wildlife Service officials report that high levels of DDT have been detected in the Gila River south of Phoenix, Arizona. What is particularly alarming is the fact that fish caught in this river have high levels of unmetabolized DDT in their tissue, which suggests that their exposure is relatively recent.**

DDT and Breast Cancer

Studies suggesting a link between breast cancer and exposure to DDT are also compelling. A prospective study of women in the New York University Women's Health Study compared serum samples taken from women who developed breast cancer six months into the study with those of women who remained cancer-free. The researchers accounted for many of the risk factors discussed in Chapter 2, including family history of breast cancer, age at first pregnancy, and whether the woman breast-fed. They found that the risk of breast cancer increased 400 percent in those women with the most elevated serum levels of DDE (DDE is the metabolite of DDT). At least three other studies have shown an association between DDT exposure and breast cancer risk.

---

*Pesticide Action Network, *Global Pesticide Campaigner* 6 (1996):4.
**Arizona Daily Star*, Wednesday, June 3, 1998.

Israel Provides a Clue

An interesting case regarding pesticide exposure (including DDT) and breast cancer comes from research that began at the Hebrew University's Hadassah Medical School in Jerusalem. It was here that researchers in 1976 began noticing that malignant breast tissue samples contained significantly higher concentrations of pesticide residues than healthy tissue samples. At the same time, other research was revealing critically high levels of pesticide residues (including DDT, lindane, and BHC) in cow's milk sold in the region. As a comparison concentrations of DDT, lindane, and BHC were 5, 17, and 100 times higher respectively than samples taken in the U.S. in the same period. Levels of BHC in human breast milk samples eventually were measured at 800 times the level of U.S. samples.*

From the 1950s until the early 1970s, these three pesticides were used liberally to fight pests in barns and cowsheds. This resulted in poisoned cows that produced contaminated milk which was then consumed by the citizens of Israel.

After public outcry, the pesticides were banned. Over the following decade the rate of breast cancer mortality dropped 30 percent. In her excellent book *Designer Poisons*, pesticide authority Marion Moses, M.D., aptly points out that it was never determined whether the women who died from breast cancer and those who remained cancer-free ever drank the contaminated cow's milk, nor were there assessments made of the blood levels of pesticides in the women with and without breast cancer. Further, there was no disclosure of other risk factors to which the women who died may have been exposed. While the reason for the decline remains uncertain, **Israel's decrease in breast cancer mortality is the only known case in which a decline has been recorded anywhere in the world.**

Pesticides as Immunotoxicants

While attention has been given to many of the health risks associated with exposure to pesticides, including their direct carcinogenicity, one area that needs much greater inquiry is the effect these chemicals have on the immune system. Based upon the data gathered so far, however, it is clear that many pesticides are immunotoxic, that is they suppress immune system function, and that in doing so, they may well heighten risk of cancer.**

---

*Richter, E.D., et al., *Environmental Research* 73 (1997):211-18.
**Exon, J.H., et al., *The Journal of Environmental Science and Health* C5 (1987):73-120.

While the immune system is extremely complex in nature, its fundamental job is to protect the health of humans and animals. It does so through a biochemical system which utilizes the bone marrow, thymus, lymphoid tissues, T-cells, B-cells, and NK-cells.

While we commonly think of the immune system as defending humans and animals from bacteria, viruses, fungi, and parasites, it also plays an important role in protecting us from cancer.* In an ideal environment, specialized cells of the immune system called natural killer cells (NK-cells), actually seek out and destroy tumor replicant cells before they become unmanageable. However, when the immune system is debilitated, as it can be by exposure to pesticides and other toxic chemicals, this protective response may be severely compromised.**

While there is yet conclusive evidence of a connection between breast cancer and chemical exposure, the data thus far should prompt strong precaution. The preponderance of evidence indicates that we may be threatening the health of every human on Earth (even the unborn), toxifying our water, soil, air, and quite possibly causing irreversible damage to the protective ozone layer. Despite this evidence, there are those who have a vested interest in perpetuating the crumbling myth that the plethora of chemicals we rely upon pose no threat "when used properly." It seems we now must ask what the "proper" use is of a substance that is a confirmed carcinogen, damages the immune system, or disrupts the endocrine system? While we struggle to answer this question, pesticide chemical use continues to climb. For example, in California, farmers increased their use of pesticides by 129 percent in just the last five years.[164] Today each of us continues to be exposed, in varying degrees, on a daily basis.

Our history is replete with cases in which, despite initial warnings of associated health problems, certain chemicals or pharmaceutical drugs were used for years, until the condemning evidence became so overwhelming it simply could not be ignored any longer. Unfortunately, rather than assume a chemical may pose a health risk until proven otherwise, we have been giving chemicals the benefit of the doubt.

---

*Steen, R.G., "Cancer and the Immune System," *A Conspiracy of Cells: The Basic Science of Cancer* (Plenum Press, New York:1993).
**Purchase, I.F.H., *Human and Experimental Toxicology* 13 (1994):17-28; Newcombe, D.S., *The Lancet* 339 (1992): 539-41.

Therefore, it seems prudent that each of us takes every precaution to avoid unnecessary exposure. Until there is concrete evidence to the contrary, we must assume that synthetic chemicals do pose a threat to our health, even though that threat may not manifest for decades after our initial exposure.

In Part II we will look at a number of strategies you can begin employing to help minimize your exposure to these substances and others.

CHAPTER SEVEN

The Stress Factor

One of the most serious consequences of mind-body interplay seen today, and therefore another major risk factor for breast cancer, is something we've come to refer to as stress. While most of us have at some time heard that stress is unhealthy, few people understand why this is so.

In Chapter 2 stress was included in the list of risk factors. This is not to say that stress is specifically associated with breast cancer or any other disease. Rather, stressful responses to life events can take a measurable toll on all of the systems of the body, not the least of which is the immune system. In addition to protecting us from opportunistic diseases such as viruses, the immune system plays an important role in protecting the body from cancer.

Current estimates are that nearly 75 percent of all visits to physicians are the result of a stress-related illness.

WHAT IS STRESS?

Dr. Hans Selye, often referred to as the "father of stress," popularized the term in the 1950s. Selye differentiated between stress, which he defined as "the nonspecific response of the organism to any pressure or demand," and the stressor, which he defined as "the stimulus, either an internal or external occurrence or event which produces the stress response." However, as we will see, it is important to remember that so-called stressors only have the potential to produce stress. Not all stressors produce stress in every individual. What is most important is our perception of the events in our lives. For example, two people are driving home in commute traffic on the same crowded freeway. While the situation has the potential to produce stress, one of these two people copes effectively with the commute, experiencing little or no stress, while the other is overwhelmed by the experience and undergoes significant emotional and physical distress. The same stressor is present for both people, yet only one experiences stress.

The stressors that we most commonly experience are associated with such events as accidents, illness, arguments, divorce, work deadlines, presentations, exams, financial burdens, and, of course, rush-hour traffic. Stressors, when responded to inappropriately, can take a significant toll on our health, leading to headaches, insomnia, ulcers, adrenal failure, high blood pressure, stroke, and heart attack. Simply put, stress can kill. Chronic stress has the effect of suppressing the function of the immune system, resulting in our being significantly more susceptible to illness and disease. In fact, **current estimates are that nearly 75 percent of all visits to physicians are the result of a stress-related illness**. To understand how a stressful experience can have such an influence on our health, it is necessary to examine a human reaction known as the stress response.

The Stress Response

The stress response, or what is often referred to as the "fight or flight" response, includes a series of physiological changes that take place in response to a perceived threat. This physiological process evolved over millions of years and now is a component of our genetic makeup. It is the legacy of the "survival of the fittest." For our ancient ancestor, the cave dweller, fight or flight was a potential lifesaver. For people today, this primitive physiological response can have grave consequences.

Consider ancient cave dwellers. At all times they were at risk of attack by wild animals. Suppose they were sitting at their fire, when suddenly a saber-toothed tiger entered the cave. In split-second timing, the cave dwellers would need to make a decision about how they would handle this uninvited guest. Essentially they had two choices: either stay and fight, or take flight and get out of the animal's way. For either choice, the cave dweller's body would be prepared for action by way of the autonomic nervous system (ANS). The autonomic portion of the nervous system regulates internal states, such as functions of the heart, blood pressure, and digestion. The ANS has two branches: the sympathetic and the parasympathetic. The sympathetic portion, the branch responsible for arousal, stimulates the stress response. In doing so, it releases powerful hormones that lead to a state of heightened arousal. Several powerful changes occur during the stress response. They include:

- Dilation of the pupils to increase visual sensitivity
- Dilation of the bronchioles in the lungs and increased rate of breathing to allow more oxygen to be transported from the lungs to the muscles
- Acceleration of the heart rate to move greater quantities of blood, and thus energy, to the larger muscles
- Tensing of the muscles to prepare for "springing" action
- Release of chemicals into the blood that will make it clot faster should there be an injury
- Breakdown of body proteins to create glucose, which instantly fuels the muscles for greater energy
- Increase in perspiration to help cool the body

All of these changes are brought about by the elevation of three hormones: norepinephrine, epinephrine (more commonly known as adrenaline), and cortisol. Their release is critical to our survival in emergency situations. However, in a non-emergency situation, where their presence is unwarranted, they can actually be toxic.

Although the possibility of having to confront a wild tiger today is highly unlikely, we all have this response programmed deep within our unconscious mind. Moreover, while today's "tigers" don't sport stripes and saber teeth, they do elicit the same stress response in many of us. Today's tigers are the stressors we discussed earlier, such as rush-hour traffic. To a greater or lesser degree, these rather common events elicit the same primitive physiological response in our body. Although they are not life-threatening, the human tendency is to react as though they were. In addition, there are some individuals who do not necessarily need a particular event to instigate this response, but live in a chronic state of elevated arousal, with tense muscles, elevated heart rate, stomach churning, chronic headaches, backaches, insomnia, sweaty palms, and anxiety.

You may be asking yourself how feelings of stress can determine whether or not you get sick. To better understand this relationship, it is necessary to examine the human immune system.

Stress and the Immune System

The immune system is fascinating and highly complex. It functions as a police force, whose job is to patrol the body in search of "non-self" invaders. These invaders, commonly referred to as antigens, may include (but are not limited to) bacteria, viruses, and parasites. As we have recently learned, an antigen does not have to be a germ or bacteria — artificial breast implants are detected by the body as "non-self" and cause immune responses in many women who have them.

The immune system is made up of a variety of highly specialized cells, each with a specific job to perform in the process of defending the body. The most common are the white blood cells. One type of white blood cell, the T-cell, helps in identifying foreign matter. Other white blood cells, known as macrophages, are programmed to recognize and ingest all antigens, as well as cellular debris. Macrophages also "present" antigens to the T-cells. Natural killer, or NK cells, are responsible for acting against tumor and virus-affected cells. NK cells locate malignant and tumor cells, attach to them, puncture holes in them, and kill them.

Research has demonstrated that the hormones released during a stress response, particularly cortisol, have the effect of suppressing the immune system by reducing the number of T-cells. The most recent discoveries in mind-body research have revealed an extremely complex network of chemical messengers known as neuropeptides. Once regarded simply as hormones, further research has revealed these communication molecules to be more sophisticated than the classic hormone or neurotransmitter. More important, these neuropeptides appear to have an even more powerful and direct effect on immune function than any of the hormones studied to date.

Research conducted by Candace Pert, former director of brain biochemistry at the National Institute of Mental Health, confirms that the mind and the nervous, endocrine, and immune systems are linked and communicate by way of tiny molecules secreted not only by the brain and immune system, but by the nerve cells of many other organs. It has been discovered that receptors for neuropeptides are highly concentrated in the areas of the brain that mediate emotion, as well as on the cells of the immune system itself.

Through immunological studies, scientists have been able to witness how our mental state can specifically affect the function of these neuropeptides and, consequently, the functioning of the cells of the immune system. States of anxiety, fear, anger, and depression, when prolonged, can have a debilitating effect on immune function. "What we see," says Dr. Joan Borysenko, former director of the Mind/Body Clinic, Harvard Medical School, "is a rich and intricate two-way communication system linking the mind, the

Those who reported the highest stress had lower levels of natural killer (NK) cells that are supposed to attack tumors.

immune system, and potentially all other systems, a pathway through which our emotions — our hopes and fears — can affect the body's ability to defend itself."

Some of the most convincing scientific evidence of this thought-chemical interplay has come from the use of Positron Emission Tomography (PET) scans. PET scans can measure cerebral blood flow and volume as well as oxygen uptake, and have enabled researchers to watch the thinking process affect these measurements. Radioimmunoassay (RIA), another highly sensitive diagnostic tool, can detect hormonal concentration changes as an individual's thoughts and appraisals of a situation change.

Volumes of studies exist on how specific events in people's lives can cause a measurable depression in the function of the immune system. Students are exceptionally qualified candidates for the study of stress and its effects, particularly when they are nearing an exam. In one study, it was found that students' T-cell response to antigens was decreased beginning six weeks prior to an exam and lasting as long as two weeks afterward. In another study, medical students approaching exam time showed a decrease of interlukin-2, another chemical component of the immune system. Interlukin-2 is critical in defending the body against cancer.

Research involving breast cancer patients conducted by psychologist Barbara Andersen and colleagues at Ohio State University, has shown that stress can have a major influence on the degree to which patients resist the disease and the likelihood that the cancer will metastasize. Testing the blood of the patients, Andersen's team found measurable effects. Those who reported the highest stress had lower levels of natural killer (NK) cells that are supposed to attack tumors.

A few studies have linked high levels of stress specifically with an elevated risk of breast cancer.[165]

Sleep deprivation is another type of stress that depresses immune function. In one study where subjects were deprived of sleep for between 48 and 77 hours, there was a marked reduction in the response of phagocytes, immune cells that normally engulf and "digest" foreign bacteria and viruses.

It has been found that chronic grieving, a more passive form of emotional stress often brought about by the loss of a loved one, can cause the same biochemical imbalance as the constant elicitation of the stress response. Consequently, this intense emotional suffering can have a dramatic effect on immune function. Most subjects who are grieving show a suppression of B-cells and T-cells, as well as a significant drop in the activity of NK cells. In one study conducted by researcher Anne O'Leary at Rutgers State University, a whopping 50 percent drop in NK cell activity was seen in bereaved individuals.

Stress is an ever-present part of modern life, and its role as a risk factor for breast cancer is becoming more apparent. In Part Two, you'll learn several techniques for minimizing stress and thus maximizing your ability to prevent breast cancer and other diseases set in motion by a weakened immune system.

CHAPTER EIGHT

Hormone-Replacement Therapy, Heart Disease, and Osteoporosis

Another crucial component to evaluating the risk factors for breast cancer is looking at the dilemma of hormone-replacement therapy (HRT). Millions of women have chosen to take postmenopausal hormone-replacement therapy out of the belief that doing so will restore qualities of youth, minimize menopausal and postmenopausal symptoms, and possibly reduce the risk of osteoporosis* and heart disease.

We know today that we can actually reverse advanced cases of CHD, and we also know that CHD is not inevitable in the first place.

While the debate over the use of HRT will continue for some time, one thing is certain, and women need to understand this: **Heart disease and osteoporosis are not caused by a deficiency of hormones. In the majority of cases, these diseases are the consequence of a lifetime of poor dietary and other lifestyle choices.** Therefore, with the correct information for making wise choices, they are largely preventable. Since HRT has been linked to a higher rate of breast cancer, rather than enter into a discussion of the possible merits and potential risks of HRT overall, this chapter looks closely at coronary artery disease and osteoporosis, and exactly what we can do

*There is no scientific evidence linking estrogen supplements to increased bone density, but only to a possible reduction in bone loss. This reduction occurs during the 5-6 year window around menopause, after which, normal bone loss resumes.

to prevent them. It is imperative that women truly understand the underlying causes of these two diseases. Hopefully the following information will confirm that there is little need to consider HRT.*

While the promise of a more youthful you is certainly seductive, again, we will see that this is not much more than a great sales pitch. Contrary to what many wish to believe, there are no "youth pills" and no ways to reverse the aging process. However, the very lifestyle choices recommended in this book can go a long way in terms of reducing the toll that age takes on our bodies and minds.

Lifestyle changes, though proven to be powerful in lowering the risk of disease, are often not considered exciting, they are not dramatic, they don't make great headlines, and they don't cost much. As a result, they don't get the attention of a culture that is fixated largely on the drama of sophisticated and expensive technology, drugs, surgery, and the like — a culture that has been deeply rooted in addressing problems after they arise rather than preventing them in the first place. In other words, our medical infrastructure is based upon disease management rather than disease prevention.

HEART DISEASE

We know that coronary heart disease (CHD) is not caused by an estrogen deficiency. Why, then, would so many doctors rush to prescribe hormone-replacement therapy, in part to lower the risk of CHD? Like osteoporosis, heart disease is a multifactorial disease. **Most of the contributing factors to heart disease are related to lifestyle choices.** We know today that we can actually reverse advanced cases of CHD,[166] and we also know that CHD is not inevitable in the first place.

Heart disease is caused by the progressive accumulation of plaque in the arterial wall. As the plaque increases, the lumen, or opening, actually becomes more narrow. Eventually, this passage can become entirely blocked, resulting in a heart attack, or, in the case of a major artery leading to the brain, a stroke.

What causes this plaque? Cholesterol and saturated fat. Where do we find cholesterol? In foods of animal origin. Anything that had a face will bring cholesterol into your diet. Plants do not produce cholesterol.

What's a safe cholesterol level? If you are over 30 years of age, 200 mg/dl is considered reasonable. Unfortunately, this is not a healthy recommendation. The reason being that the average heart attack victim has a cholesterol value of 240 mg/dl, and the average American, 205 mg/dl. Yet people have

*To address symptoms of menopause using natural progesterone cream, see Dr. John R. Lee's *What Your Doctor May Not Tell You About Menopause* (Warner, 1996).

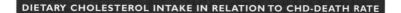

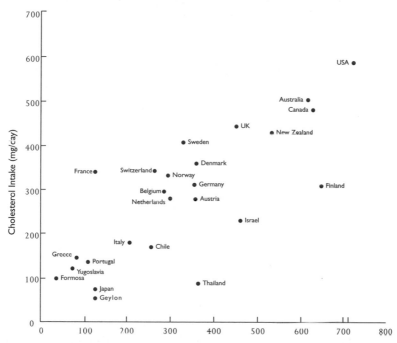

DIETARY CHOLESTEROL INTAKE IN RELATION TO CHD-DEATH RATE

CHD-related death rate per 100,000 male pop. (Age 55-59)
SOURCE: Connor, W. *Preventive Medicine* 1 (1972): 48-83.

heart attacks all the time at 200, 190, and 180. But there is a threshold. In the Framingham heart study, which has been going on for 40 years, it was found that 150mg/dl is virtually a guarantee of freedom from heart attack. In this study, not one person with a cholesterol value of 150 has ever suffered a heart attack. I set out years ago to meet a goal of 150. By practicing the strategies outlined in this book, I not only met this goal but also surpassed it. I reached 116mg/dl. With the rare exception of a genetic predisposition, such as hypercholesterolemia, in which cholesterol levels soar to over 300 even in childhood, each of us has the potential to bring our cholesterol down to what it would have been as a healthy teenager.

Reducing the risk of CHD primarily comes from changing our diet. Secondarily, we can reduce our risk further through aerobic exercise. Finally, we can further cut our risk through stress-reduction strategies such as meditation. I will address all three of these ways of reducing the risk of CHD in Part Two, because all three of them also work to lower the risk of breast cancer.

KEY RISK FACTORS FOR CORONARY HEART DISEASE (CHD)

- High cholesterol diet
- High-fat diet
- High blood pressure
- Sedentary living
- Stress

OSTEOPOROSIS

Osteoporosis is the name for a disease that results in an increasing narrowing and frailty of the bones, ultimately resulting in bone fractures. It is a significant problem for Americans, and **each year some 1.5 million such fractures are reported, 500,000 of which occur in premenopausal women**. Fractures occur most frequently in the hip, rib, wrist, and vertebrae. In advanced cases, a mere sneeze can result in a fractured rib.

Today an American woman has a 40 percent risk that she will suffer a bone fracture in her lifetime. Some 20 percent of those who suffer a hip fracture and undergo surgery die within 18 months. Why is this happening? Conventional wisdom holds that the osteoporosis we see in America is a consequence of calcium deficiency. As you will see, this is not the case.*

CAUSE OF OSTEOPOROSIS

Calcium deficiency is not the cause of osteoporosis any more than hormone deficiency is the cause of coronary heart disease. Instead, osteoporosis is a consequence of calcium losses. Despite a severely compromised diet, most Americans manage to consume plenty of calcium. Unfortunately, we don't retain that calcium where we would like: in our bones. Several factors contribute to calcium losses, all of which I will present here. One of the most important, research indicates, is an excessive intake of animal protein.

High-Protein Diets Cause Bone Loss

We covet protein in America. Not only do we eat an enormously protein-rich meal three or more times a day, but many of us also consume protein supplements in the form of powders, pills, and "energy bars." Currently, there is a resurgence of fad diet books touting the virtues of a high-protein diet. Judging from book sales, Americans are eating up this nutritional lore. Today, the average total protein intake is huge, sometimes exceeding 400 percent of our actual needs. Can too much of a good thing be bad? You bet!

---

*While calcium is a key player, there are many other nutrients essential to bone health. Please see Alan R. Gaby, M.D.'s book, *Preventing and Reversing Osteoporosis* (Rocklin: Prima Publishing, 1994).

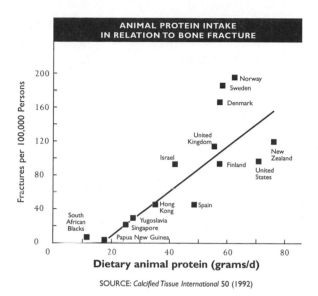

SOURCE: *Calcified Tissue International* 50 (1992)

While protein is an essential nutrient, the fact is that the human body needs an exceptionally small amount to perform all its tasks. The World Health Organization has estimated that protein needs to total only about 4 percent of our total daily caloric intake. Yet some Americans are consuming far in excess of this, and they are paying a heavy price for doing so.

When the body's protein needs have been met, protein excesses make the blood, which is normally kept in a balanced alkaline state, become more acidic. To buffer this rise in acidity, the body draws upon calcium stores. Most of the calcium in the body is stored in the bones. Therefore, to buffer the blood acidity, the body leaches calcium from the bones. If this calcium leaching were to occur very infrequently, it might not pose such a problem. However, when one regularly consumes a high-protein diet, calcium is being robbed from the bones around the clock, resulting in a chronic, silent degeneration of bone.

Research has shown that as long as one's protein intake remains high, bone loss will continue unabated, regardless of how much calcium one consumes.[168] In other words, it doesn't matter how many Tums you eat or how many calcium supplements you take. **If you keep flooding your body with protein, you will keep dissolving your bones.** Many people believe that all they need to do is take more calcium. If more calcium were the key, the native Inuits would have the strongest bones on earth. As noted earlier, they eat upwards of 2,500 mg of calcium every day, and they have the highest rate of osteoporosis in the world![168] Because of their dependence upon animal flesh (walrus, seal, fish, and whale meat) as a food source, the native Inuits consume some 400 grams of protein daily. This protein excess is their problem.

Animal Protein Is Worse

While protein excesses will cause calcium losses, the leaching process is exacerbated by proteins found in animal products. In fact, **research has shown that by age 65, women who have followed a meat-centered diet have lost 35 percent of their bone mass, whereas women who have followed a plant-centered diet have lost on average 18 percent of their bone mass.**[169]

Osteoporosis is not a problem in parts of the world where protein is consumed in moderation, particularly if it is derived from plant sources. Even when protein is eaten beyond one's needs, when the protein is derived from plant sources, the leaching process is minimized.[170] **It has been suggested that simply moving to a vegetarian diet could cut calcium losses in half in the average American.**[171]

Consider the women in China who labor well into their eighties carrying rice bags and tools all over fields and hillsides. They have strong bones, they don't eat dairy products, and they are not on hormone therapy. This may be largely due to the fact that they are not sedentary, they use their bones through weight-bearing exercise, and they don't eat a high-protein, meat-centered diet or other foods that rob the bones of calcium, namely, foods high in protein, phosphorus, and caffeine. Also, they don't smoke.

What About Milk Mustaches?

The popular ad campaign that shows a slew of celebrities posing with a supposed residue of milk on their upper lip, indicating, of course, that they drink milk, might lead one to believe that cow's milk is not only an admirable "habit of the glamorous," but perhaps the answer to America's osteoporosis epidemic. A recent study regarding calcium and osteoporosis made national headlines. The study warned that Americans are plagued by osteoporosis and that the cause of this epidemic is simply that Americans are "passing by the dairy case."[172] **To suggest that this country's problem with osteoporosis is a consequence of not drinking the milk of another species is to abandon all common sense. Does it make any sense that for humans to fulfill their calcium need they should essentially nurse from cows for the rest of their lives?** The thought is preposterous (but deeply ingrained in our culture). Further, our fixation on calcium derived from cow's milk suggests that there are no other sources of dietary calcium. This is far from the truth. (Please see Chapter 8 for calcium sources).

Refined Grains and Bone Health

Prior to being processed and refined, whole foods contain an abundance of important nutrients for not only bone health but also health in general. However, when foods are processed to make them more shelf stable or visually appealing, their nutritive value is seriously compromised. Consider, for example, wheat flour. In its whole form, this grain is a nutritional powerhouse, but when it is refined, stripped of its important bran, and bleached into white flour, it loses 80 percent of its magnesium, 60 percent of its calcium, and 50 percent of its manganese — three minerals essential to bone health. Think about all the flour products you eat regularly, from sandwich bread, crackers, and cookies, bagels, donuts, muffins, and pastries to the pasta that you buy at the supermarket and virtually any pasta that you are served in a restaurant, to pancakes and waffles and other grain-based foods. In most instances, you are probably eating refined, nutrient-depleted flour products. The price of eating these nutritionally valueless foods is the osteoporosis epidemic in this country.

Sodium and Bone Health

Most people are familiar with the fact that a diet high in sodium is not healthy. Most of the attention has been focused around sodium's propensity to increase blood pressure. Yet sodium also plays a negative role in bone health. Diets high in sodium cause the bones to dissolve more quickly. A diet high in sodium and high in protein provides a double whammy. It has been estimated that one high-sodium, high-protein, low-calcium fast-food hamburger can lead to a loss of 22 mg of calcium.[173]

Phosphorus and Bone Health

Excessive levels of phosphorus exacerbates the problem of calcium losses. Foods high in phosphorus and low in calcium, such as red meat, make calcium absorption difficult and thereby elevate the risk of osteoporosis.[174] Again, with regard to meat, we get the double-whammy of a load of excessive protein and phosphorus at the same time. A dependence upon carbonated soft drinks, which are high in phosphorus, also contributes to the problem of osteoporosis.

Sugar and Bone Health

In addition to all its other problems, sugar exacerbates calcium losses and therefore contributes to risk of osteoporosis. Sugar interferes with calcium absorption, and leads to elevated production of hydrochloric acid, making the body increasingly acidic. As mentioned, the body prefers an alkaline state and therefore must buffer that acidity, ultimately drawing on calcium to do so.

Smoking and Bone Health

Smoking causes bone loss. A woman who smokes a pack a day in her adulthood can expect to lose up to 10 percent additional bone mass by menopause. Smoking takes its toll on bone by dosing the body with cadmium, nicotine, lead, and other toxic substances.

Caffeine and Bone Health

Caffeine delivers more than a "rush" to the user. In addition to raising cholesterol and taxing the adrenal glands, this widely used stimulant causes the body to excrete calcium in the urine. With the average American drinking 43 gallons of coffee a year, we are getting our fair share of caffeine, even before considering sodas, teas, chocolate, and the many common medications that contain caffeine. Studies have shown that the more caffeine one consumes, the more calcium one will excrete in the urine. One study showed that two cups of coffee can result in the loss of 15 mg of calcium. Another study found that women who consume four cups of coffee a day triple their risk of hip fracture compared to women who drink little or no coffee.[175] In fact, hip fracture risk goes up markedly with caffeine consumption.[176]

Fluoride and Bone Health

Chapter 6 mentioned the health hazards associated with consuming fluoride from drinking water. Suffice it to say that fluoride is far too dangerous for any of us to be consuming. In addition to its numerous other problems, many studies have shown fluoride intake is clearly associated with elevated risk for hip fracture.[177]

Exercise and Bone Health

Have you ever broken an arm or a leg and had the limb in a cast for a few weeks or months? Remember how the muscle looked when the doctor finally removed the cast? Chances are the muscle had atrophied to a size disproportionate to the other limb. Like muscles that have been isolated in a cast and have shrunk, bones become frail with disuse. For bones to remain strong, they need to have weight bearing on them. When there is no weight placed on bones, the bones are not stimulated and they begin to demineralize. Fortunately, a little bit of exercise can help shrunken muscles regain their size and strength. Similarly, with bones, it takes weight-bearing exercise to restore their proper strength.

We have learned a good deal about bone health from the space shuttle missions. In fact, space physiologists at the National Aeronautics and Space Administration (NASA) have determined that their astronauts may lose bone mineral at a rate of 1 percent to 1.5 percent a month. The mineral depletion occurs mostly in the hip and lower spine. One former astronaut, Dr. Norman E. Thagard, lost 11.7 percent of his bone mineral during an extended 115-day stint in space in 1996.

In one study, a program of weight-bearing exercise increased bone mass in subjects by 5 percent in as little as nine months.[178] One of the most encouraging studies confirming the role of exercise in increasing bone mass was conducted by researchers at Queen Elizabeth Hospital in Toronto, Canada. After only one year, subjects showed a bone mass increase of a whopping 8 percent.[179] **Even 80-year-old women have increased their bone mass with as little as 30 minutes of exercise three times a week.**[180]

Women who consume four cups of coffee a day triple their risk of hip fracture compared to women who drink little or no coffee.

Since her diagnosis of breast cancer in 1982, Ruth Heidrich, author of *A Race for Life*, has won over 700 trophies and medals for marathon and triathlon competitions. What may be even more impressive is, despite a family history of osteoporosis, she has consistently increased her bone mass since her forties. Today, at age 63, she retains a bone mass greater than the average 30-year-old American woman.* Her secret is regular exercise combined with a vegan diet.[181]

---

*The average 30-year-old female has a peak bone density (PBD) of 411 mg/cm^2 (centimeter squared). At age 50 Dr. Heidrich's PBD was 447 mg/cm^2. At age 60 it was 466 mg/cm^2.

Exercise is the key to keeping bones strong. The more stress we subject a bone to, the greater the bone's response in strengthening. Researchers at Johnson Space Center have developed and are testing an array of exercise equipment they hope can be used in future trips to space, including a special bicycle built for two. Because we live in a gravity environment, all we need do is move our bodies by walking, jogging or running, or step-climbing.

Women who are more active not only have stronger bones but also suffer fewer fractures.[182] **Individuals who exercise regularly have a bone mass that is as much as 27 percent greater than those who are sedentary.**[183] Athletes are even better off, with bone mass as much as 50 percent greater than non-athletes. Even noncompetitive runners in their sixth and seventh decade of life have been shown to have bone mass 40 percent greater than their same-aged sedentary counterparts.[184]

KEY RISK FACTORS FOR OSTEOPOROSIS

- Excessive animal protein
- Tobacco
- Alcohol
- Cigarette smoke
- Caffeine
- Sugar
- Fluoride
- Lack of exercise
- Refined grains

So, you see, osteoporosis is no mystery at all. With the average American eating a high-protein, meat-centered diet loaded with sodium, refined grains depleted of their important minerals, and foods with calcium-binding preservatives, consuming some 800 phosphoric acid-containing soft drinks a year, and getting little exercise to stimulate the skeletal system, it follows logically that we are faced with this epidemic. The great news is that each of us can positively affect all of these risk factors through simple lifestyle changes, and these same lifestyle changes can also reduce the risk of breast cancer.

PART TWO

Preventing Breast Cancer:
The Seven-Step Prevention Plan

"The doctor of the future will give no medicine, but instead will interest his patients in the care of the human frame, in diet, and in the cause and prevention of disease."

Thomas Edison

CHAPTER NINE

The Revised American Diet™

Since mammography is clearly not an effective way to prevent breast cancer (it can only diagnose it), just how can women go about reducing the risk of the disease? It's obvious that several of the risk factors listed earlier are beyond your control. There is, after all, nothing you can do about your height, sex, race, or other hereditary traits, and there is nothing you can do about the age at which you reached menarche. However, you can do something about other risk factors. For instance, depending on your age and life circumstances, you may be able to decide whether and when you will become pregnant, whether you will breast-feed, and whether you will choose hormone-replacement therapy after menopause. As previously mentioned, depending on your age, you may even be able to influence when you reach menopause by following a low-fat, high-fiber plant–centered diet.

In addition to possibly having some control over some of the factors just mentioned, you can exert even more control with regard to other lifestyle choices. For example, you can abstain from alcohol, avoid cigarette smoke, avoid toxic chemicals, and minimize exposure to radiation. You can also reduce stress and the toll it takes on your immune system through regular exercise and meditation. In this chapter, we will explore one of the most powerful ways you can reduce your risk of breast cancer: improving your diet. In subsequent chapters in Part Two, we'll also discuss other factors in greater detail, beginning with diet (and related topics) and concluding with stress-reduction techniques.

DANGEROUS RECOMMENDATIONS

A spokesperson for Burger King fast-food restaurants once said, **"If someone wants to cut . . . fat, they can order their Whopper without mayonnaise."**[185] Unfortunately, despite the constant message we receive from industry and from the health-care associations, if we are truly serious about reducing risk of disease, it's going to take a bit more than skipping the mayonnaise. When American hospitals are inviting McDonald's fast food franchises to set up shop in their wards,[186] and when the public health associations are dispensing advice that is contrary to a preponderance of international scientific and epidemiological evidence about diet and disease, we can no longer be surprised at the state of the average American's health.

Consider the fact that the current national dietary guidelines, which are endorsed and recommended by the American Heart Association, American Cancer Society, American Dietetic Association, and the American Medical Association, suggest a cholesterol intake of no more than 300 mg a day and a fat intake of 30 percent of total calories. Then consider the fact that one in two Americans will develop heart disease, and one in three will develop cancer in their lifetimes, and things are getting worse. Clearly, the prevailing recommendations are not helping.

As already indicated, studies have shown that the superfluous designation of 30 percent of calories as fat and 300 mg of cholesterol offer no protection against cancer or heart disease. On the contrary, a mountain of research has shown that such a recommendation is not only ineffective but leads to disease.

How do we maximally reduce risk of disease via diet? The most effective way is to move toward a plant-centered diet. Doing so will sharply reduce our intake of saturated fat and total fat, cholesterol, pesticide residues, and other contaminants. Doing so will at the same time sharply increase our intake of protective dietary fiber, vitamins, minerals, and phytochemicals.

I want to stress that what I am proposing is not another fad diet but a comprehensive change in the type and quantity of foods you consume. In the following pages you will find guidelines and suggestions for following the Revised American Diet.™ If you follow these guidelines, you will reap many rewards that will last a lifetime, including reducing your risk of breast cancer.

When you make the transition from a diet that is centered on contaminated, high-fat animal products to a diet centered on whole grains, vegetables, legumes, and fruits, you need not be concerned with percentages and grams per serving calculations because the recommended foods are significantly lower in fat, have moderate levels of protein, and contain no cholesterol. They are also naturally high in complex carbohydrates. Whole grains, vegetables, legumes, and fruits are all nutrient-dense, meaning they naturally contain higher levels of the micronutrients (vitamins and minerals), important phytochemicals, and beneficial fiber our body needs. The types of food you choose to eat — not the exact measurement of such foods — make a desirable nutrient balance possible. Weighing foods, counting calories, and calculating fat grams per serving become things of the past.

The point of this book is to show you how best to reduce your risk of breast cancer. In addition, the lifestyle choices outlined in this book happen to be those that can also significantly reduce your risk of heart disease, stroke, hypertension, diabetes, osteoporosis, and kidney disease.

Two of the most important protective constituents of a plant-based diet are fiber and phytochemicals.

THE ROLE OF FIBER

Dietary fiber is a group of carbohydrate substances that compose the cell walls of plants such as fruits and vegetables, whole grains, and nuts and seeds. There are a variety of types of fiber, including cellulose, hemicellulose, gums, pectins, and lignans, each of which acts in a different way. Although fiber is resistant to digestion, it performs many roles, such as increasing fecal bulk, lessening transit time (time for digestion and elimination), and reducing cholesterol levels.

For the past decade, we have heard about the wonders of fiber. Yet most of what we have heard regards its role in weight management and protection against colon cancer and heart disease. The reality is that **a host of other diseases and conditions are strongly related to a low-fiber diet, including diabetes, varicose veins, constipation, diverticulitis, obesity, and gallbladder disease. Fiber is also essential to protecting against breast cancer.**[187]

Fiber confers protection from breast cancer for several reasons. The first is that high-fiber foods, such as fruits, vegetables, and whole grains, are significantly lower in fat content than the high fat-foods that prevail in the Standard American Diet (SAD). By eating foods that are rich in fiber, we displace those that are high in fat.

Fiber protects in another important way. It has been shown that fiber lowers risk of breast cancer by reducing the level of circulating hormones in the body.[188] After hormones have fulfilled a particular assignment in the body, they are sent to the digestive tract, where, if conditions are favorable, they are escorted out of the body. Specifically, the hormones are bound with fiber and then excreted in the feces.[189] However, in the event that insufficient fiber is available, this process can be hampered, and the hormones can be reabsorbed into circulation and heighten risk.[190] **In a large study of Canadian women, it was found that women at the highest fifth of dietary fiber intake had a breast cancer risk 30 percent lower than those women at the lowest fifth.**[191]

As previously mentioned, Asian nations have a much lower rate of breast cancer than the U.S. Their fat intake (particularly animal fat) is significantly lower, since their diet is based largely on plants, which are rich in fiber.

If you watch television during prime time, you will likely see a variety of commercials for various fiber supplements. These supplements are intended to remedy the fact that the standard American diet (SAD) is largely deficient in natural fiber. The simple reason is that the SAD is centered around animal products — beef, chicken, pork, fish, dairy products, etc. — none of which contain any fiber. Fiber exists only in plant foods. Because the SAD is so deficient in fiber, the average American ingests at best 10 to 20 grams of fiber daily. However, in countries where colon cancer, heart disease, and breast cancer are only a fraction of that seen in America, fiber intake ranges from at least 33 grams to as high as 70 grams a day!

THE ROLE OF PHYTOCHEMICALS

It is well known that those who eat four to five servings of fruits and vegetables a day have about half the incidence of cancer of the general population. Aside from providing high levels of fiber, fruits and vegetables offer certain compounds responsible for reducing the risk of cancer: phytochemicals. Sometimes called nutriceuticals, phytochemicals have been shown to have anticancer properties. Some actually detoxify carcinogens, while others prevent carcinogens from penetrating cells. Still others prevent malignant changes from occurring in cells that have already been exposed to carcinogens (see phytochemical table).

Consider genestein. This phytochemical, which is abundant in soy foods, has been shown in over 30 studies to be a powerful tool in disrupting the cancer cascade. Specifically, research has shown that genestein inter-

	EXAMPLES OF FIBER-RICH FOODS
FRUITS	Apples, bananas, berries, cantaloupe, grapefruit, guava, mangoes, oranges, pineapple, papaya, pears.
VEGETABLES	Artichoke, broccoli, Brussel sprouts, carrots, corn, cauliflower, kale, potatoes, spinach, squash.
WHOLE-GRAINS	Whole wheat bread, muffins, bagels, and tortillas. Bran, bran-muffins, oatmeal, shredded wheat cereal, whole grain pasta, Bulgar wheat, buckwheat, barley, quinoa, amaranth, millet, triticale, popcorn, rice cakes
LEGUMES	Black beans, lima beans, kidney beans, navy beans, yellow, red, and green lentils, pinto beans, split peas, black-eyed peas, fava beans.

feres with angiogenesis,[192] the process whereby new blood vessels are established. Without these vessels bringing in oxygen and nutrients, the tumor is effectively starved to death. Currently, the National Cancer Institute is spending enormous sums of money to further research two cancer drugs, angiostatin and endostatin, which have been shown to effectively eradicate tumors in mice.[193] These drugs operate on the very same principle as genestein: depriving tumors of their own blood supply.

Researchers at the University of California at Berkeley have demonstrated that another phytochemical, indole-3-carbinol, found in abundance in broccoli, halts the growth of breast cancer cells in culture.

Leonard F. Bjeldanes, professor of toxicology in the College of Natural Resources at UC Berkeley says, "What's exciting about this is that indole-3-carbinol is a very effective agent against mammary tumors —it's one of the most effective agents at blocking tumorigenesis in rats. Given in the diet, indole-3-carbinol can block 95 percent of all mammary tumors in rats." It is believed that the compound works by demoting the production of the recently discovered enzyme CDK6 (cyclin-dependent kinase 6) which is involved in regulating cell division.

While broccoli is certainly one of the superstar-foods in terms of prevention, indole-3-carbinol is also found in cabbage, Brussel sprouts, bok choy, kale, chard, and turnips.

Tangeretine, a flavanoid found in tangerines, has been shown to be one of the most potent anticancer compounds. **In the case of breast cancer, tangeretine is believed to fortify E-cadherin, which can be thought of as a wall that prevents cancer cells from invading breast cells.**[194] In cancer, E-cadherin is usually inactive or produced in insufficient quantities. A diet

PHYTOCHEMICALS AND THEIR SOURCES		
PHYTOCHEMICAL	ACTION	SOURCE
ALLYLIC SULFIDE	Fortifies cells to better detoxify themselves, prevents proliferation of tumor cells, enhances immune function and reduces cholesterol levels; cancer protection associated with breast, mouth, skin, colon	Onion, garlic, leeks, chives, shallots
CAPSAICIN	Neutralizes carcinogens	Hot peppers
DITHIOLTHIONES	Prevents cancer by activating enzymes that prevent damage to DNA	Broccoli, cabbage, collards
ELLAGIC ACID	Tumor inhibition; Eliminates reactive oxygen and other free radicals	Strawberries, cranberries, blackberries, walnuts
GENESTEIN	Prevents initiation of hormone–dependent cancers—breast, prostate, ovary, cervix; may prevent metastasis of tumors by preventing them from forming new capillaries	Legumes, seeds, soybeans, licorice
INDOLES	Promotes anti-cancer enzymes and helps neutralize "fake estrogen" created by toxic chemicals	Brussels sprouts, cabbage, cauliflower, collards
ISOTHIOCYANATES	Protects DNA from damage; Inactivates phase 1 enzymes that activate carcinogens; promotes phase 2 enzymes that inhibit carcinogenesis	Brussel sprouts, cabbage, kale, radishes, turnips, watercress
LIGNANS	Interferes with estrogen synthesis, thereby reducing risk of breast uterine, and cervical cancer	Flaxseeds, whole grains, legumes, walnuts, seeds
LYCOPENE	Antioxidant action prevents the initiation of cancer	Tomatoes, watermelon
MONOTERPENES	Transports carcinogens out of cells before cells turn cancerous	Oranges, lemons, limes
PHYTIC ACID	Interferes with free radical production and inhibits tumor growth	Whole grains, legumes, fruits, vegetables
PHYTOSTEROLS	Prevents cancer promoting hormones from binding to receptor cites of sensitive tissues; Protection associated with breast, prostate, and colon cancer	Whole grains, legumes, carrots, parsley, soy foods, yams
PROTEASE INHIBITORS	Inhibits action of the cancer–promoting enzyme protease; may help mitigate the effects of radiation	Soy foods, legumes, nuts, tomatoes
SAPONINS	Inhibits cancer–promoting enzymes and halts cancer cell multiplication	Soy foods, legumes
SULFORAPHANE	Inhibits tumor growth; helps anti-cancer enzymes eliminate carcinogens; Protection associated particularly with breast cancer	Broccoli, Brussel sprouts, cabbage, kale turnips, collards

that supplies tangeretine could change that. These are just a few superstars singled out from a host of some several hundred phytochemicals that may be providing significant protection to those who consume a fruit- and vegetable-rich diet.

Because they may compete with endogenous estrogen, phytoestrogens, weak estrogens produced in some plants, are also important in breast cancer risk reduction. It is thought that the protection may be derived when these plant estrogens bind to estrogen cell receptors on cells, and effectively block the more powerful estrogens made in the body. Soy foods are abundant in phytoestrogens.

OTHER BENEFITS OF THE REVISED AMERICAN DIET™

Increased Energy

Who couldn't use more energy throughout the day? Invariably, people who make the transition to a low-fat diet that is high in complex carbohydrates find they have increased energy levels. There are a couple of reasons for this. First, because of their high fat content, meats, eggs, and dairy products require a longer period of time to be digested. Digestion requires a good deal of energy, energy that is unavailable to other processes during this period. Consequently, one may feel slow and lethargic after a high-fat meal. Moreover, contrary to popular belief, high-fat animal products are a poor source of energy. In fact, they are very low in carbohydrates. Complex carbohydrates are the best source of fuel for the body. Whole grains, vegetables, legumes, and fruit are the best sources of energy.

	CARBOHYDRATE COMPARISON	
FOOD	Serving	Carbohydrates
BAKED POTATO	3 $^1/_2$ oz.	25 grams
Pork Loin		0 grams
PINTO BEANS	3 $^1/_2$ oz.	26 grams
Chicken Breast		0 grams
WHOLE-WHEAT SPAGHETTI	3 $^1/_2$ oz.	28 grams
Cheddar Cheese		1 gram
DATES	3 $^1/_2$ oz.	74 grams
Milk		5 grams

Easy and Permanent Weight Loss

It's doubtful that you are reading this book in order to learn how to manage your weight, but lasting weight loss is another one of the perks that come from following a low-fat, high-fiber diet. As mentioned previously, research has continued to show that as body weight increases, so does the risk for breast cancer.

The FDA currently lists nearly 30,000 diets. At any one time, it is estimated that 65 million Americans are on some form of weight-loss diet, whether it be one promoted in a fashion magazine or one promoted at one of the thousands of weight-loss centers around the country. This year, Americans will spend $35 billion on weight–loss programs.[195] This is a clear indication of how confused and unsuccessful people are when it comes to controlling their body weight. If any of these diets worked and comprised a healthy and safe way of eating, there would be no market for the other 29,999 diets. Some diets, such as liquid protein, are life-threatening, resulting in heart arrhythmia, which can even lead to death.

Many fad diets that prescribe extremely low-calorie and/or carbohydrate intake do see rapid weight loss. However, the loss is generally in lean body mass (muscle and water), as well as in glycogen stores. Unfortunately, many people will misinterpret this fat loss when they step on their scale. In 95 percent of cases, after a restrictive fad diet, the body regains the lost weight. What is worse is that the weight is regained not in the form it was lost (muscle and water), but as fat!

When an individual significantly drops his or her calorie consumption, the body moves to a state of alert. No, you won't hear bells and whistles going off, but inside changes are occurring. In fact, the body interprets this reduction in calories as potential starvation. If starvation is "just around the corner," what do you think your body will do to prepare? That's right, conserve! The body shifts into "survival mode" and begins to slow the metabolism, burning fewer calories (up to 15 percent less) and holding on to fat reserves as a way of assuring itself a lasting supply of energy. Essentially, it operates with less. This is why dieters say, "At first the weight dropped off like magic, then suddenly I couldn't lose a pound." While this safety mechanism is a wonderful response to actual starvation, it is extremely frustrating for someone attempting to lose weight. Even though fat cells may shrink to a degree (the number of fat cells stays the same), they are very sensitized and "anxious" to gain back what they lost after a short-term diet ends. In fact, research has shown that **with each successive diet a chronic dieter fol-**

lows, not only does she regain more weight more easily but also her meta-bolic rate (the rate at which her body utilizes calories) continues to slow further each time. Furthermore, people who are on calorie-restricted diets don't feel well. They feel deprived of food, lack energy, and become irritable.

What is the solution to this madness? Simply, reduce your fat intake, not your calorie intake. Our bodies are highly complex organisms that are conducting thousands of processes an hour. To carry out all these tasks — not to mention fuel our daily activities — energy is required, and energy comes from food. Massive cutbacks in calories mean massive cutbacks in energy and dysfunction on all levels. When you eat a diet that is low in fat, rich in whole grains, and high in fiber, it is not another temporary diet. It is not something you begin a few weeks before the senior prom, before a day at the beach, or when trying to fit into a particular outfit. It is a way of life, a comprehensive change from the Standard American Diet (SAD).

Much of the struggle with weight that many people experience is the result of the types, not the quantity, of food they eat. To illustrate, each gram of fat yields nine calories, while a gram of either carbohydrate or protein has only four. Consequently, on a traditional high-fat diet, you consume exces-sive amounts of calories before achieving a feeling of satiety and before sat-isfying the body's nutritional needs. On the RAD, however, when eating whole grains, vegetables, legumes, and fruits, which are naturally low in calories, you can actually eat more without gaining weight. You simply cannot feel deprived of food on a low-fat diet. **You would need to consume over 15 cups of brown rice before you would take in as much fat as in a single cup of whole milk, and over 50 cups of broccoli before equaling**

FOOD	FAT COMPARISON	
	Serving	Fat
BANANA	3 $1/2$ oz.	1 gram
Ground Beef		21 grams
BROWN RICE	3 $1/2$ oz.	1 gram
Roasted Ham		21 grams
BAKED POTATO	3 $1/2$ oz.	0 grams
Cheddar Cheese		33 grams
OATMEAL	3 $1/2$ oz.	1 gram
Pepperoni		39 grams

the amount of fat in a cheeseburger. Imagine eating 50 bananas. Impossible, right? Yet that's what you would have to do to get the same amount of fat in an average 12-ounce steak. Or, choose between 97 baked potatoes or one plate of fettucine Alfredo. Furthermore, while excessive fat is easily stored by the body, excess carbohydrates cannot be stored directly by the body and most go through a conversion process whereby 23 percent of the calories are utilized. Finally, complex carbohydrates actually increase your metabolism!

Consider that some 4 billion people living on this planet today have eaten a plant-centered diet all their lives, and most of them have no problem with maintaining a desirable body weight. They don't count calories, fat grams, or percentage of calories as fat, and they certainly aren't worried about being in some "euphoric zone." It's the types of foods they eat that enable their carefree and successful diet and the numerous health benefits they enjoy.

Controlled Insulin Production

Insulin is a hormone produced by the pancreas and released in the body to help balance blood sugar. The greater the amount of sugar released in the blood, the more insulin is necessary to remove the sugar and transport it to waiting cells. Unfortunately, once blood sugar levels drop, two things happen: Energy levels are lowered, so that one feels tired, and appetite increases. With an increase in appetite comes an increase in eating. So, it makes sense that to help control our appetite and maintain a more stable supply of energy, we need to maintain lower levels of insulin.

The refined carbohydrates and high-fat foods found in the Standard American Diet lead to increased insulin production. This is one reason why average Americans can never seem to get enough food. When they ingest refined foods such as white flour, sugar, and many other sweets, the sugar content enters their blood very rapidly, raising blood sugar levels too fast. The opposite effect occurs when they eat whole, unrefined foods found in the Revised American Diet.™ These foods are largely complex carbohydrates and contain significant amounts of fiber. They are assimilated by the body more gradually than refined foods. For this reason, less insulin production is required, and a roller-coaster appetite is avoided.

Lowered Blood Pressure

Although the human body can function on 500-1,000 mg of sodium daily, in reality the Standard American Diet contains somewhere between 3,000 and 6,000 mg a day. An excess of sodium plays an important role in high blood pressure. Chinese physicians wrote about this in 1000 B.C. in the Yellow Emperor's Classic of Internal Medicine, saying, "Excess of salty flavor hardens the pulse." It works like this: When the body is over-whelmed with sodium, it begins to retain water. Consequently, the volume of blood being transported in the body increases. The blood vessels auto-matically compensate by contracting, thereby reducing blood flow. However, this compounds the problem, as the heart is required to work even harder to move the blood through the narrowed blood vessels.

FOOD	SODIUM COMPARISON	
	Serving	Sodium
STRAWBERRIES	1 cup	1 mg
Ham	3 oz.	1,203 mg
ZUCCHINI	1 cup	3 mg
Hot Dog	4 oz.	1,146 mg
BROCCOLI	1 cup	17 mg
Blue Cheese	1 cup	1,884 mg
BROWN RICE	1 cup	5 mg
Parmesan Cheese	2 oz.	950 mg

Lowered Blood Cholesterol

An elevated cholesterol level is a strong predictor of heart disease and stroke. Average Americans eat in a way that predisposes them to a 50 per-cent chance of suffering a heart attack sometime in their lives. The primary reason is that average Americans eats large amounts of cholesterol as well as saturated fat, which stimulates the liver to manufacture cholesterol. When you eliminate animal products from your diet, however, you elimi-nate all sources of cholesterol and a good deal of the saturated fat, and your blood cholesterol level will drop significantly.*

*For a detailed discussion of cholesterol levels and risk of heart disease, please see Chapter 8.

FOOD	CHOLESTEROL COMPARISON	
	Serving	Mg
ALL GRAINS	1	0 mg
Egg		275 mg
ALL VEGETABLES	3 1/2 oz	0 mg
Goose		96 mg
ALL FRUITS	3 1/2 oz	0 mg
Sour Cream		116 mg
ALL LEGUMES	3 1/2 oz	0 mg
Chicken Breast		85 mg

COMMON QUESTIONS ABOUT A PLANT-BASED DIET

Often when one considers making the transition to a plant-based diet, questions arise about a few nutrients and whether such a diet can sufficiently provide for them. Most often the concern is over adequate protein, iron, vitamin B_{12}, and calcium.

Will I Get Enough Protein?

Protein may well be the most overrated nutrient there is. This is particularly so in the West. Probably the key reason as to why protein gets such overemphasis in the diet is that it is largely mistaken as an energy nutrient. That is, most people believe that protein consumption equates to energy. The more one eats, the more energy they will have, so goes the logic. This simply is not the case.

This idea may have gained popularity as far back as the mid-1800s, when a physiological chemist named Leibig suggested that muscular energy came from oxidized protein. Although it was learned by the mid-19th century that such was not the case, that in fact carbohydrates and fat are the chief fuels for muscular energy, and the body spares protein so that it can be utilized foremost in the construction and maintenance of body tissues, hormones, enzymes, and antibodies, the myth has persisted until today, and the obsession with getting enough protein rages on.

Are Americans finding themselves with little energy during their day? By and large, lack of energy is a common complaint in Americans. Yet, as indicated in the last chapter, a protein deficiency is simply not the cause.

In fact, protein deficiency is virtually unheard of in America. Americans consume as much as 400 percent of their protein needs, and, as indicated earlier in Chapters 4 and 8, the price is high: accelerated calcium losses leading to osteoporosis, heightened risk of cancer, and overworked kidneys leading to kidney disease. The canary in the coal mine, so to speak, is the fact that 20 million Americans suffer from kidney damage, and some 200,000 live with the assistance of an artificial kidney machine. Can you guess what one part of the protocol is for treating kidney patients? If you guessed a low-protein diet, you're correct. One of the first things done is to place the patient on a low-protein diet. The prescription works quite well, too. According to Dr. Ping H. Wang, assistant professor of medicine at the University of California at Irvine, at least five studies of patients suffering from chronic kidney disease "show a 30 percent reduction in complications with a low-protein diet."

Getting Enough Protein Is Easy

Getting enough protein in the diet is much easier than most people have been led to believe. The reality is that as long as Americans eat sufficient calories to maintain their body weight, and derive them from a variety of whole grains, legumes, vegetables, and fruits, they will do just fine. The idea that one needs to combine foods in some precise order at a certain time to meet protein requirements is simply a myth of the past. In fact, one would be hard pressed to find a documented case of protein deficiency in the United States. **According to a U.S. Department of Agriculture study, even when following a vegetarian diet, Americans consume on average 150 percent of their protein requirement.**

How Much Protein Do We need?

Consider that in infancy, a time at which the body is developing very rapidly and when the protein needs are the greatest they will ever be, nature provides about 5 percent of calories as protein in the form of mother's milk. Still, to be absolutely sure and to compensate for any number of conditions that may exist, human protein requirements have been calculated higher by a variety of organizations. Although the World Health Organization recommends 4.5 percent of calories as protein, the Food and Nutrition Board of the U.S. Department of Agriculture recommends 6 percent of calories as protein. The National Research Council recommends 8 percent of calories as protein.

The World Health Organization states, **"There are no known advantages from increasing the proportion of energy derived from protein . . . and high intakes may have harmful effects in promoting excessive losses of body calcium and perhaps in accelerating age-related decline in renal (kidney) function."**

A glance at the table below will confirm that plant foods are quite abundant in protein.

Percent	PERCENT OF PROTEIN IN PLANT FOODS
	VEGETABLES
49%	SPINACH
40%	CAULIFLOWER
34%	PARSLEY
28%	ZUCCHINI
24%	CUCUMBER
18%	TOMATOES
11%	POTATOES
47%	BROCCOLI
38%	MUSHROOMS
34%	LETTUCE
26%	GREEN BEANS
21%	CELERY
16%	ONIONS
	LEGUMES
43%	TOFU
26%	KIDNEY BEANS
23%	CHICK PEAS
29%	LENTILS
26%	NAVY BEANS
30%	GREEN PEAS
	GRAINS
20%	RYE
16%	OATMEAL
11%	BARLEY
17%	WHEAT
15%	BUCKWHEAT
8%	BROWN RICE

What About Iron?

We have always been told that we need to be sure to get adequate iron in our diet, particularly women who lose iron through menstruation. Iron is essential to the formation of blood cells, the transport of oxygen and the maintenance of tissues. Yet too much iron, as pointed out earlier, can be problematic, raising risk of heart disease and, as some recent research suggests, Parkinson's disease. Like protein, however, most people get plenty of iron without thinking about it. The reason is that most Americans follow a meat-centered diet, and meat is a rich source of iron. Plant foods also offer plenty of iron, although in more moderate amounts than meats, and studies have shown that individuals following vegetarian diets do just fine in meeting their iron needs.[196]

IRON CONTENT OF VARIOUS FOODS (mg per 1 cup)	
SPINACH	6.4 mg
PINTO BEANS	5.4 mg
WHOLE WHEAT FLOUR	5.2 mg
CHICKPEAS	4.9 mg
SOYBEANS	4.9 mg
BARLEY	4.2 mg
LENTILS	4.2 mg
PEAS	3.4 mg
PUMPKIN	3.4 mg
RAISINS	3.0 mg

Where Will I Get Vitamin B_{12}?

Vitamin B_{12} is made by microorganisms that occur in soil and fermented foods. Today, the primary sources of this vitamin are animal products and possibly some fermented foods. Although the human need for B_{12} is curiously small (0.1-2 mcg), and there have been reported only a handful of deficiency cases, it plays an important role in both nerve function and blood cell growth and should not be ignored.

There are a couple of options for assuring adequate B_{12} in the diet. The most obvious is to take a supplement. Another option is to consume cereals, certain soy-based foods such as meat analogues and soy milks, that have been fortified with the vitamin. Persons who prefer a supplement should look for a reputable brand of vegetarian-based B_{12} with a dosage of 3 mcg and should take the supplement three times a week.

By following the standard American diet, most people consume several hundred times their B_{12} need daily and have sufficient stores to last them months or even years. Vitamin B_{12} deficiencies in the U.S. are rare, and in almost all cases reported, they are not due to inadequate intake but to the body's reduced ability to absorb the nutrient with age.

Sources of Vitamin B_{12}

- Nutritional yeast (Red Star T-6635+)—(marketed as Red Star Vegetarian Support Formula)
- Kellogg's Nutri-Grain Cereal
- Healthy Choice Just Right Cereal
- Eden Soy Extra Soy Beverage
- Fortified textured soy protein

Is There Sufficient Calcium in a Plant-Centered Diet?

A good deal has already been said about calcium and fulfilling our needs easily by following a plant-based diet. As further reassurance, a study conducted to determine the nutritional adequacy of 119 strict vegetarians (vegans) found that the average calcium intake was 825 milligrams a day — 325 milligrams more than the World Health Organization (WHO) recommends. This was without any dairy products or supplements.[197] This well exceeds the WHO's recommended daily intake for calcium. **In a 1984 USDA survey, the National Food Consumption Survey, vegetarians were shown to have calcium intakes that exceeded those of the general population, at all ages.**

Certain foods are particularly rich in calcium, and they certainly should be a regular part of your diet. As always, the key in deriving all of the nutrients our body needs is in eating a broad variety of whole foods. See the table below for examples.

Do I Need to Take Supplements?

There is also the question of supplementation. "Should I take supplements?" I often am asked. My position on supplements is as follows. **Ideally, vitamins, minerals, fiber, and phytochemicals and other so-called superfoods are best derived from whole, unrefined natural foods. This gives us the nutrients and compounds in what can be thought of as balanced chemistry, the way in which nature intended**. However, nature

mg per 1 cup	CALCIUM CONTENT OF VARIOUS FOODS
	VEGETABLES
245 mg	SPINACH
197 mg	TURNIP GREENS
177 mg	BROCCOLI
158 mg	CHINESE CABBAGE, COOKED
148 mg	COLLARD GREENS
147 mg	DANDELION GREENS
115 mg	RHUBARB
104 mg	MUSTARD GREENS
102 mg	SWISS CHARD
94 mg	KALE
57 mg	ONION
	LEGUMES
175 mg	SOYBEANS
144 mg	TEMPEH
128 mg	NAVY BEANS
100-320 mg	TOFU
95 mg	PEAS
90 mg	GREAT NORTHERN BEANS
86 mg	PINTO BEANS
55 mg	LIMA BEANS
47 mg	BLACK BEANS
37 mg	LENTILS
	ANIMAL FOODS
115 mg	MILK
16 mg	BEEF STEAK
14 mg	EGG
14 mg	CHICKEN
11 mg	PORK
10 mg	TUNA
	NUTS AND SEEDS
245 mg	ALMONDS
209 mg	HAZELNUTS
131 mg	PISTACHIOS
126 mg	SUNFLOWER SEEDS
110 mg	SESAME SEEDS

never intended for humans to be drinking water and breathing air containing cancer-causing agents like chlorine and the dry–cleaning solvent perc, and carbon tetrachloride. Nor does nature account for the conventional farming practices that have left much of the farm soil in the U.S. deficient of nutrients. In light of increasing scientific evidence and because of the degree to which we are exposed to toxic chemicals in our air, water and foods, I believe that a degree of supplementation is warranted. Some factors, such as our increasing exposure to ultraviolet radiation (due to deterioration of the protective ozone layer), ionizing radiation (via X-rays), and second-hand smoke, heighten cancer-promoting free radicals. Other factors, such as food preservatives, black tea, synthetic fats, and prescription drugs, can interfere with the absorption of certain vitamins and minerals that are essential to preventing cancer. Finally, despite our intention to eat the most wholesome foods, we sometimes eat foods that are nutritionally inferior because of cooking procedures that are out of our control (for example, in restaurants and on airplanes), or because of growing, processing, and storage and transportation procedures. Consider that irradiated foods, which are creeping into the marketplace, quietly but surely, are depleted of a number of vitamins, including up to one-third of their vitamin C, due to the irradiation process.[198] So, regardless of what diet and lifestyle one follows, I believe that some supplementation is warranted.

Antioxidants

There is a good deal of evidence that supports taking vitamins C (1000-2,000 mg/day) and E (400 iu/day), and selenium (100 mcg/day). Vitamins C, E, and selenium not only boost the immune system, they are also powerful antioxidants, playing an important role in disarming free radicals and thus helping to prevent cancer.[199]

Vitamin C

The volume of studies confirming the protective effect of vitamin C supplementation is enormous. Epidemiological studies have shown us that a high intake of vitamin C will reduce the risk of most cancers by about 50 percent.[200] Vitamin C protects against radiation-induced cellular damage and inhibits the formation of cancer-causing nitrosamines (derived from nitrite-containing cured foods).[201] Vitamin C is found in fruits and vegetables.

Vitamin E

Like vitamin C, vitamin E is a powerful antioxidant. Research has shown that women with lower blood levels of vitamin E and selenium have a higher risk of developing breast cancer.[202] Vitamin E supplementation has been shown to boost immune function,[203] reduce the likelihood of early onset dementia, prevent cataracts,[204] and reduce damage caused by exposure to ultraviolet light and radiation.[205] Vitamin E is found in whole grains and nuts.

Selenium

Selenium is increasingly recognized as an essential component in cancer prevention.[206] This mineral has been shown to boost antioxidant enzyme levels in cells and to help mitigate the damage caused by exposure to radiation.[207] Selenium stimulates the immune system and increases the number and activity of white blood cells, particularly the natural killer cells (NK) that are responsible for searching out and destroying cancer cells.

In a recent study, researchers at the University of Arizona found that a daily supplement of selenium decreased the risk of a variety of cancers by up to 60 percent. Selenium does its work synergistically working closely with vitamins C and E to combat free radical production. While selenium is normally found in abundance in grains, garlic (its presence in garlic may be one reason the food is considered protective), and asparagus, due to conventional farming practices, our soils in the U.S. have become quite depleted of the mineral.

Acidophilus

Acidophilus is a collective term for important bacteria that live in the intestines. This healthful flora has many roles, including assisting in the production of B vitamins, keeping harmful bacteria in check, and even helping prevent the formation of carcinogenic compounds. Since 30 percent of the immune system is in the digestive tract, intestinal health is essential to proper immune function. Also, in order to most fully derive the health-protective nutrients from the foods you eat, your intestines—specifically healthy intestinal flora—need to be in good health. Healthy intestinal bacteria can be depleted by alcohol consumption, antibiotics, and cigarette smoke. Few Americans have not taken at least one course of antibiotics in their lifetime. Antibiotics do a fine job of eliminating unhealthy bacteria in the body. However, they do so in an indiscriminate fashion, managing to eliminate the healthy flora that keep our digestion and assimilation of foods

VITAMINS AND THEIR SOURCES				
	VEGAN SOURCES	BENEFITS	U.S.R.DA	DEPLETES/INHIBITS
A (pro-vitamin beta carotene)	Carrots, sweet potatoes, pumpkin, broccoli, winter squash, cantaloupe, papaya, peaches, beets, parsley, spinach, apricots, Swiss chard, garlic, spirulina	Prevents night blindness. Helps resist infection. Maintains integrity of epithelial membranes. May reduce risk of cancers of the breast, lung, prostate, and cervix, as well as heart disease. Acts as an antioxidant, reducing damage caused by free radicals in the body.	5,000 I.U. No RDA exists for beta carotene	Coffee, excessive iron
B₁ (Thiamine)	Whole grains, peanuts, sunflower seeds, soy, beans, fruits, vegetables	Assists in carbohydrate metabolism, maintenance of nerve tissue, appetite and digestion. Essential to normal function of nervous tissue.	1.5 mg	Tobacco, alcohol, coffee
B₂ (Riboflavin)	Almonds, whole-wheat bread, leafy greens, legumes	Prevents anemia, cataracts. Plays role in formation of enzymes. Assists in light adaptation.	1.7 mg	Tobacco, alcohol, coffee
B₆ (Pyridoxine)	Citrus fruits, peppers, leafy greens, cauliflower and potatoes	Prevents anemia and nerve damage. Facilitates utilization of tryptophan and other amino acids. May reduce risk of neural tube defects in the fetus.	2.0 mg	Tobacco, alcohol, coffee, birth control pills, radiation
B₁₂ (Cobalamin)	Miso, tempeh, nutritional yeast, spirulina, fortified cereals, and soy foods	Prevents anemia. Essential to normal development of red blood cells. May reduce risk of heart disease and nerve damage.	2.0 mg	Tobacco, alcohol, coffee, laxatives
Biotin	Mung beans, lentils, brown rice, whole grains, brewer's or nutritional yeast	Promotes growth; important to fat, carbo-hydrate, and protein metabolism; hair and skin	0.3 mcg	Alcohol, coffee
Folicin (Folic acid)	Leafy green veggies, root veggies, whole grains	Required for cell growth and division; formation of red blood cells	0.4 mg	Tobacco, alcohol, coffee
Niacin (Nicotinic acid)	Beans, rice bran, green vegetables, whole wheat, nuts	Promotes growth; maintenance of nervous system; maintenance of skin, digestion; protein, fat and carbohydrate metabolism.	20 mg	Alcohol, coffee
Pantothenic acid	Orange juice, legumes, whole grains, mushrooms	Protects skin; supports adrenal glands; antibody production	10 mg	Alcohol, coffee
C (Ascorbic acid)	Rose hips, strawberries, green peppers, citrus, leafy greens, tomatoes, Swiss chard, broccoli, asparagus, oranges	Acts as an antioxidant, reducing damage caused by free radicals. Prevents scurvy. Helps wounds heal. Facilitates absorption of iron. Helps maintain resistance to infection. May reduce risk of cancer and heart disease.	60 mg	Tobacco, antibiotics, aspirin, cortisone
D	† Sunshine	Prevents bone deformation. Facilitates absorption of calcium. May help in preventing osteoporosis.	5 mcg	Mineral oil
E (Tocopherol)	Wheat germ, cold pressed oils, leafy greens, oatmeal, brown rice, nuts and seeds, whole grains	Acts as an antioxidant-reducing damage caused by free-radicals. Prevents anemia. May reduce risk of heart attack.	30 I.U.	Rancid oil, chlorine, birth control pills

SOURCE: Food and Nutrition Board, National Academy of Sciences—National Research Council. U.S.R.D.A revised, 1989.
*Beta carotene is not a vitamin, but a pro-vitamin found in certain foods. When metabolized by the body it is converted to vitamin A.
† Vitamin D is actually not a vitamin but a hormone the body synthesizes when the skin is exposed to sunlight. All the vitamin D we need can be obtained through 15 minutes of sun exposure a day. After a summer of sun exposure, the liver will store enough vitamin D to last through the winter months. Those who live in Northern climates and see little sunshine or are confined to the indoors would be wise to consume vitamin D-fortified soy milk or take a supplement.

g = gram   mg = milligram   mcg = microgram   I.U. = international units   1,000 mg = 1 gram   1,000 mcg = 1 milligram

	MINERALS AND THEIR SOURCES			
	U.S.R.D.A	VEGAN SOURCES	DEFICIENCY SYMPTOMS	FUNCTIONS	DEPLETES/ INHIBITS
Calcium	800 mg 1,200 mg. (preg/lact)	Leafy green vegetables, broccoli, collards, kale, almonds, tofu, fortified soy products, lentils, raisins, navy beans, sesame seeds	Brittle bones, heart palpitations, muscle pain, tooth decay	Required for development and maintenance of bones and teeth. Important to blood clotting, nerve transmission, heart rhythm, and contraction and expansion of muscles.	Excess protein, caffeine, magnesium deficiency
Chromium	None established	Whole-grain cereals, corn oil, brown rice potatoes, brewer's yeast	Retarded growth, atherosclerosis	Enhances insulin function; stimulates enzymes in metabolism of energy; important in synthesis of fatty acids, cholesterol, and protein.	None
Cobalt	None established	Leafy greens vegetables, fruits	Retarded growth, pernicious anemia	Maintains red blood cells; functions with vitamin. B12; activates some enzymes.	None
Copper	2 mg	Soybeans, raisins, nuts, legumes, molasses, avocados, raisins, oats	Skin sores, impaired respiration, general weakness	Important in function of enzymes; with Vitamin C it forms elastin; formation of red blood cells; hair and skin, bone formation	Excessive levels of zinc
Iodine	150 mg	Mushrooms, iodized salt, kelp, onion, garlic, spinach, carrots	Irritability, dry hair, nervous dysfunction, cold hands and feet	Regulates energy production and rate of metabolism; prevents goite; promotes healthy hair, skin, nails.	None
Iron	10 mg (males) 15 mg (females)	Cherry juice, molasses, wheat germ, leafy green vegetables, shredded wheat, dried fruits, legumes	General weakness, anemia, constipation	Important to formation of hemoglobin and myoglobin; promotes protein metabolism; promotes growth.	Excessive levels of zinc
Magnesium	350 mg (males) 280 mg (females) 350 mg (preg/lact)	Molasses, whole grains, nuts, kelp, bran, green vegetables, seeds, oats	Muscular excitability, nervousness, tremors	Catalyst in the utilization of protein, fats and carbohydrates, phosphorus, calcium. Assists in maintenance of arteries, heart, and nerves.	None
Manganese	None established	Whole grains, nuts, legumes, leafy greens, bananas, celery, pineapple, bran	Hearing loss, dizziness	Enzyme activator; maintains sex hormone production, tissue respiration, skeletal development.	Excessive intakes of phosphorus and calcium
Phosphorus	800 mg 1,200 mg (preg/lact)	Legumes, nuts, whole grains; sesame, sunflower, and pumpkin seeds; garlic	Weight loss, appetite suppression, fatigue, nervousness	Works with calcium to maintain bones, teeth; cell growth and repair; heart muscle contraction; nerve activity	Excessive intakes of magnesium, aluminum, and iron
Potassium	None established	Whole grains, legumes, sunflower seeds, dried fruit, peaches, nuts, molasses, bananas	Respiratory dysfunction, poor reflexes, dry skin, nervousness, irregular heartbeat	Controls activity of heart muscle, nervous system, and kidneys; growth; muscle contractions.	Coffee, diuretics, alcohol, cortisone, laxatives
Selenium	None established	Broccoli, onions, bran, wheat germ, tomatoes, brown rice, brewer's yeast, whole grains	Premature aging, heightened cancer risk	Beneficial for kwashiorkor; works with vitamin E; preserves tissue elasticity Antioxidant.	None
Zinc	15 mg (males) 12 mg (females)	Soybeans, brewer's yeast, spinach, legumes, mushrooms, sunflower and pumpkin seeds	Delayed sexual maturity, inhibition of taste, suppressed appetite, fatigue, retarded growth	Assists in digestion and metabolism of protein, carbohydrates and phosphorus; component of insulin; prostate gland function	Phosphorus deficiency, alcohol

optimal. For example, it has been shown that the body's ability to assimilate the important phytochemicals found in soy foods is dependent upon healthy intestinal flora.[208] When good bacteria are killed-off, the population of fungi and yeast (especially candida) that have been kept in check, can grow dramatically. If this bacteria spreads sufficiently, it can result in fatigue, severe digestive problems, and allergic reactions. Acidophilus supplements can help restore natural intestinal bacteria, enabling better digestion and assimilation of foods, protecting against bad bacteria, and support immune function.

Choosing Supplements

While a basic vitamin/mineral supplement is a wise idea, most provide Vitamins C, E and the mineral selenium in minimal amounts. Therefore, you may wish to purchase individual supplements of these. Look for a reputable brand of vitamin C in 500 or 1,000 mg tablets or capsules (smaller dosages will require swallowing more tablets). Take 500-1,000 mg early in the day and one late in the day, with meals. Vitamin E and selenium should also be taken together with meals. Be sure your Vitamin E is the natural form (d-alpha-tocopherol). This is better recognized and assimilated better by the body. Acidophilus supplements should be taken according to the manufacturer's suggestion.

NOTE: Supplements are not a license to skip meals or make poor food choices. They are a form of insurance. Women planning a pregnancy should consult their physician about a good prenatal vitamin/mineral formula as a form of insurance, in addition to their whole foods diet.

SUGGESTED SUPPLEMENT PROGRAM

Vitamin C 1,000-2,000 mg/day
Vitamin E 400 iu/day
Selenium 100 mcg/day
*Acidophilus 1-2 capsules daily (see manufacturer's dosage suggestion)

For the many benefits outlined in this chapter, shifting from the Standard American Diet (SAD) to the Revised American Diet™ (RAD) is the single most powerful thing you can do to reduce your risk of breast cancer. In Chapters 19-21, we'll explore in detail the different foods of the Revised American Diet™ and how to begin to incorporate these foods.

---

*Periodic supplementation contingent upon intestinal health and use of antibiotics and alcohol.

CHAPTER TEN

Going Organic

If you are truly motivated to protect your health and sharply reduce your risk of breast cancer as well as other cancers, you will want to make the effort to purchase organically produced fruits, vegetables, and grains at every opportunity. You will also want to choose, whenever possible, organic nuts, seeds, herbs, spices, and the foods made with them. There is simply too much evidence that indicates that the agricultural chemicals that are routinely used to treat foods are toxic to humans, and some are deadly. In Chapter 6, we reviewed some of the worst threats posed by the overuse of pesticides in our country and abroad. It is crucial that we do what we can to avoid these toxic chemicals.

Conventionally grown strawberries, according to FDA inspection data, are laced with more endocrine-disrupting pesticides than any other food.

Every time that you choose conventionally farmed foods over organic, you are increasing your cumulative exposure to chemicals and raising your risk of disease. **If you follow a conventional diet, it is estimated that you will consume about 150 mcg of pesticides each day.**[209] Yet, this does not have to be so. The fact of the matter is that there is no "acceptable level" of intake of a toxic chemical that is a carcinogen, has hormone-disrupting potential, or causes neurological damage. Moreover, each time we choose conventionally grown foods over organics, we are supporting the continued poisoning of our nation's soil, air, and water, a toxic legacy that will be a burden for generations to come.

In addition to the multitude of *legal* toxic chemicals that are routinely used on fruits, vegetables, grains, and other foods, *illegal* chemicals (deemed so presumably because the degree to which they are toxic to humans is beyond the limits of tolerability) have been detected in the American food supply. In a review of 14,000 records of the Food and Drug Administration's pesticide-monitoring program, researchers at the Environmental Working Group identified 356 illegal uses of pesticides.[210] **In their review of the data, they found that 24.7 percent of peaches, 15.7 percent of pears, 12.5 percent of apple juice, and 12.4 percent of blackberries** *contained illegal pesticides, and 11.7 percent of green onions were found to have illegal pesticides used on them.* Remember, all conventionally grown produce is subject to the application of legal toxic pesticides.

PESTICIDE KARMA

Some of the more deadly pesticides that have been banned from use within the United States are still manufactured in the U.S. and then exported for use in foreign countries. The bulk of them end up being applied to crops in South and Central America. Between 1992 and 1994, over 45 million pounds of restricted pesticides known to have "very high toxicities and environmental hazards" were exported for use outside the United States.[211] Since 1944, the U.S. has exported nine tons of U.S.-banned pesticides and some 40 million pounds of pesticides that are known hormone disruptors.[212] In addition to the disturbing fact that we are knowingly manufacturing a chemical that poses a severe threat to humans, animals, and the environment, is the imminent return of this toxic cargo on the very fruits and vegetables that we increasingly import to U.S. markets. To allow this is to sanction the slow poisoning of Americans, as long as the poison is being applied outside U.S. borders. As an example, **chlordane, a pesticide banned in the U.S. but exported from the U.S. all over the world, has been detected on fish, rice, mushrooms, squash, and beef that is imported into the U.S.**[213]

While some supermarket chains have attempted to assure their customers that their produce is free of "detectable residues," random samplings confirm that such promises simply cannot be kept. For example, Richard Wiles of the Washington, D.C.-based Environmental Working

Group, examined **data for a three-year period and found that over 80 percent of peach, apple, and celery samples contained residues of one or more pesticides. As many as eight different pesticides were detected on a single apple.**[214] **Among the detected residues, 12 known carcinogens, 17 neurotoxins, and 11 pesticides that interfere with the endocrine and reproductive systems were identified.** A more recent Food and Drug Administration (FDA) study found pesticide residues in 48 percent of the random samples of fruits and vegetables.[215]

Moreover, the latest research indicates that a number of the most commonly used pesticides have endocrine-disrupting properties, and among populations where there is the most extreme exposure to such chemicals through groundwater, breast cancer rates are very high.[216]

For example, Vinclozolin, an anti-androgenic pesticide is commonly used on cucumbers, grapes, lettuce, onions, bell peppers, raspberries, strawberries, tomatoes, and Belgian endive.[217] In fact **conventionally grown strawberries, according to FDA inspection data, are laced with more endocrine-disrupting pesticides than any other food.**[218]

Some pesticides, such as the soil fumigant methyl bromide, threaten human and animal health in a more indirect manner. Some 350 pounds of this poison gas is used per acre to grow strawberries. The U.S. Environmental Protection Agency classifies methyl bromide as a "Category-1 Acute Toxin" (the highest risk assessment level) because it is known to cause severe poisonings that can result in neurological damage and reproductive harm. The unique hazard of this gas is that it is a powerful destroyer of the protective ozone. So great is methyl bromide's threat to the ozone that 295 atmospheric scientists have concluded that the most significant action that can be taken to protect the ozone is to eliminate all dependence upon this agent.* As the ozone is further depleted, rates of ultraviolet-induced skin cancer (now striking 1 in 105 persons) and cataract blindness continue to soar the world over.

Currently the FDA manages to test only a fraction of the foods in the U.S., and its current analytical methods are only sensitive enough to detect one-third of the more than 600 pesticides in use today.[219]

WHAT ARE ORGANIC FOODS?

Organic foods have been grown without the use of harmful synthetic chemical pesticides, and fertilizers. For a food to be certified organic, it must

---

*Funding A Better Ban: Smart Spending on Methyl Bromide Alternatives in Developing Countries (San Francisco: Pesticide Action Network, 1997).

have been grown on farmland that has been free of such chemicals for a minimum of three years. The mere fact that a particular process hasn't detected a chemical residue is not an indication of the food's having been grown organically. If a food is truly organic and free of harmful chemicals, it must be deemed so by proper posting and certification stickers.

When foods are grown using conventional farming methods, they are subjected to enormous quantities of harmful chemicals, many of which have not been tested for safety and some of which are established human carcinogens. In California alone, 400 million pounds of farming chemicals are used annually. **According to a report by the National Academy of Sciences, chemical pesticides may cause an additional 1.4 million cases of cancer in this generation of Americans.**

NOT JUST SAFE — NUTRITIOUS

Studies have shown that foods grown organically have a greater nutritional value than conventionally grown foods.[220] At Rutgers University, researchers studied the mineral quality of conventional produce and organic produce and discovered that, on average, the organically grown foods had an 87 percent higher content of magnesium, potassium, manganese, iron, and copper. Organic tomatoes were found to yield 500% more calcium than conventional tomatoes.[221]

HOW TO KNOW IT'S ORGANIC

Of the 28 states that have organic farming regulations, only 16 currently require certification. In these states, farmers of organic foods must be certified by either the state or a private certification agency that has been accredited by the U.S. Department of Agriculture.

Certified organic foods will usually have a sign nearby indicating that they are organic. Some fruits and vegetables bear a small certification sticker as proof. If you are buying from a farmer's market, the definition can sometimes become blurry. In this case, ask the vendors for some official documentation that the foods they are selling are indeed organic.

Some markets may provide food designated as "transitional." This term applies during the period leading up to certification. Although synthetic pesticides are typically not used on such produce, the soil it is grown in has not been pesticide-free for the required three-year period for certification. So while the produce may not yet have the stamp of approval, it should be safer than any conventional produce.

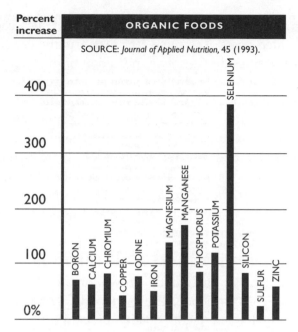

Percentage increase of important minerals found
in organic foods over those grown conventionally.

Some foods are more vulnerable to pests than others and, consequently, tend to receive a greater degree of pesticide applications. The following graph depicts the degree to which common foods are treated with pesticides relative to strawberries, which are considered to be the most pesticide-contaminated of fruits and vegetables. In addition to having the greatest numbers of different residues detected (up to 30 different pesticides have been detected on strawberry samples), in a recent survey, strawberries were found to have the greatest residues of endocrine-disrupting chemicals.[221]

The following chart was produced by the Center for Science in the Public Interest utilizing data from the FDA, compiled and analyzed by the Environmental Working Group. Since strawberries have the worst level of pesticide residues of any food, they are designated "100" and used as a comparison in assessing the level of pesticide residues of other common foods.

In addition to eating more of the healthy foods described in Chapters 20 and 21, making the commitment to purchase organic foods is a crucial component in lessening your risk of breast cancer. And the more consumers join you, the sooner organic foods will become more affordable. Given their anticancer properties, they are already a bargain.

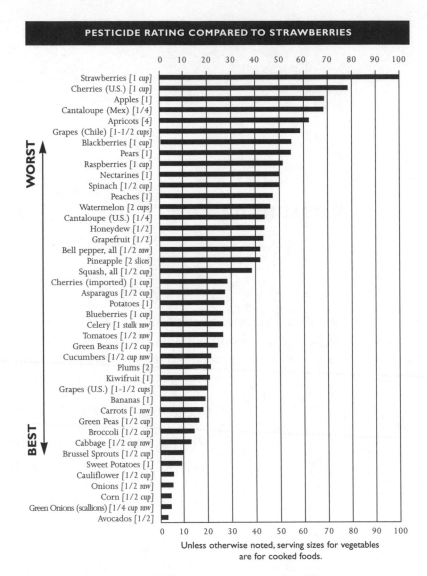

PESTICIDE RATING COMPARED TO STRAWBERRIES

Strawberries [1 cup]
Cherries (U.S.) [1 cup]
Apples [1]
Cantaloupe (Mex) [1/4]
Apricots [4]
Grapes (Chile) [1-1/2 cups]
Blackberries [1 cup]
Pears [1]
Raspberries [1 cup]
Nectarines [1]
Spinach [1/2 cup]
Peaches [1]
Watermelon [2 cups]
Cantaloupe (U.S.) [1/4]
Honeydew [1/2]
Grapefruit [1/2]
Bell pepper, all [1/2 raw]
Pineapple [2 slices]
Squash, all [1/2 cup]
Cherries (imported) [1 cup]
Asparagus [1/2 cup]
Potatoes [1]
Blueberries [1 cup]
Celery [1 stalk raw]
Tomatoes [1/2 raw]
Green Beans [1/2 cup]
Cucumbers [1/2 cup raw]
Plums [2]
Kiwifruit [1]
Grapes (U.S.) [1-1/2 cups]
Bananas [1]
Carrots [1 raw]
Green Peas [1/2 cup]
Broccoli [1/2 cup]
Cabbage [1/2 cup raw]
Brussel Sprouts [1/2 cup]
Sweet Potatoes [1]
Cauliflower [1/2 cup]
Onions [1/2 raw]
Corn [1/2 cup]
Green Onions (scallions) [1/4 cup raw]
Avocados [1/2]

WORST

BEST

Unless otherwise noted, serving sizes for vegetables
are for cooked foods.

SOURCE: Environment Working Group and the Nutrition Action Health letter,
Center for Science in the Public Interest

CHAPTER ELEVEN

Consuming Pure Water

Not only is it important to consume pure food if you want to reduce your risk for breast cancer, it is also important that you drink pure water. Water is indisputably the most important and predominant nutrient in your body. While you could survive for up to a month without food, you would perish in only days without water. Three-quarters of the human body weight is made up of water, so it is no wonder that we must constantly replenish our water supply to keep the body functioning properly. Water assists in many vital functions. It

Consuming purified water is another step you can take toward reducing the risk of breast cancer.

helps in the assimilation of foods and vitamins, carries nutrients and oxygen to the cells, and acts as a vehicle for the removal of body wastes. Therefore, water is a purifier. Probably the most important job water has in the body is regulating body temperature.

While it is recommended that the average person consume between eight and ten glasses of water each day, depending on diet and daily activities, regular strenuous exercise increases one's water needs because of the amount of water lost through perspiration. An individual can perspire as much as a quart of water per hour while training on a hot day. During exercise, our muscles generate heat, causing the body temperature to rise. In a very efficient process, heat from the muscles is removed by water present in the bloodstream and brought to the skin surface, where it is released by way of perspiration. As this process continues, the body eventually becomes dehydrated and is no longer able to effectively cool itself. In a state of dehydration, the amount of water normally contained in the blood drops low enough to create a drop in blood volume. In response to this drop, the body automatically constricts the blood vessels leading to the skin, serving to prevent a drop in blood pressure. You probably guessed the next phase. That's right. With a reduction of blood reaching the skin comes a reduction of heat being dissipated through the skin. The result? You overheat! And contrary to what we assume, thirst is not an accurate indicator of our water needs. You can avoid this risk simply by keeping your body well hydrated as you exercise.

By no means should you try to consume a large quantity of water all at once. Not only is it difficult, but for some, it's sickening. The best method is to consume six to eight glasses of water a day even if you are not exercising. Prepare a large pitcher of water with a little fresh lemon squeezed into it, and over the course of the day, try to drink a glass or two every couple of hours. At work, keep glass-bottled water close at hand. Before a workout, it's a good idea to drink about one cup of water. Then, every 10 to 15 minutes (depending on how vigorously you are exercising), consume another three to four ounces. Remember, you needn't be hot to lose water. The body loses water through the vapor of breath. In cold weather, the kidneys increase urine production, which also contributes to dehydration.

WATER FILTRATION

In Chapter 6, we looked at the sea of chemicals awash in our water, including such toxic chemicals as fluoride, lead, and chlorine. All told, the EPA says, "More than 740 million pounds of toxic chemicals pour into waterways annually, in addition to tons of other pollutants ranging from used motor oil to raw sewage."[223] Nobody concerned about their health should be drinking from or bathing in this toxic soup! Consuming purified water is another step you can take toward reducing the risk of breast cancer.

Many people have chosen to purchase bottled water to protect themselves against lead and other pollutants. While some brands offer nothing other than partially treated tap water, several reputable national brands print both the source and the chemical nature of their water. Buying bottled water at the supermarket can become expensive, however, and the accumulation of plastic bottles is harmful to the environment, and as indicated earlier, may pose a serious risk to human health because of the release of endocrine-disrupting chemicals. For quality and value, your best option is to install a water purification system in your home, allowing you to save on bottles and/or delivery costs while protecting the environment and your health. Let's look at a few of the different "point-of-use" filtration systems available to learn which might be your best choice.

Carafe Filter

Because they are affordable and need no installation, carafe filters are very popular. Unfortunately, these portable filtration systems are also the least effective way to purify your water. As the name implies, this system is composed of a carafe with two internal compartments. Water is poured into the top compartment and slowly trickles through the filter and into the lower compartment. While such a system may cost only $25 to $35, it has a maximum capacity of one gallon and requires 20 minutes to provide minimal filtration. Unfortunately, carafe systems are not effective at much other than reducing the poor taste and odor of tap water.

Solid Carbon Block

Solid carbon filtration effectively removes bad tastes and odors, chlorine, THMs, asbestos, lead, and most pesticides, as well as giardia and cryptosporidium. Small units can be mounted to faucet heads for as little as $25. Countertop systems begin at $225. Whole-house systems can be purchased for between $400 and $800. A word of caution: Carbon filters should be replaced according to the manufacturer's recommendation. Carbon filters that are not changed promptly can easily breed harmful bacteria.

Distillation

With the exception of volatile organic compounds (VOCs) which evaporate easily, distillation will remove just about every pollutant you should be concerned about, including arsenic, cadmium, chromium, iron, lead, giardia cysts, nitrates, and sulfates. In this system, water is brought to a boiling point. The purified water is turned to vapor, then condensed to a liquid again and stored in a holding container. All substances that can not evaporate are retained in a holding chamber. In addition to being highly effective, there are no filters to be replaced on distillers. Systems cost between $200 and $900 for countertop models and between $800 and $4,000 for whole-house systems. The disadvantages of a distillation system are that it requires electricity to operate and it removes most of the beneficial minerals in water. Then again, if you follow the dietary guidelines outlined in Part Three, this becomes a moot point. Also, distillation is extremely slow, requiring up to seven hours to purify a gallon of water. If your water needs are high, it probably is not the right choice.

Reverse Osmosis

Reverse osmosis (R.O.) removes most contaminants found in water, including asbestos, radioactive elements, toxic metals, and fluoride, with the exception of chlorine. Although this system is wasteful, using three to six gallons of water to produce one gallon of purified water, it is by far the most thorough. Reverse osmosis should be your choice if your drinking-water supply contains high levels of lead. An R.O. system is the most effective means to filter lead, removing 98 percent to 99 percent in most cases. Some systems combine a reverse osmosis filter system with an activated carbon "post-filter" that acts to catch any remaining organic chemicals that pass by the R.O. filter, including chlorine. This combination is hard to beat. Models range in price from $399 to $1,500. Note: R.O. systems are vulnerable to clogging if water is particularly mineral-rich. It is essential that you have the quality of your water analyzed and that your dealer know your water quality prior to selling you an R.O. system. R.O. systems are fairly complex to install and will likely require professional assistance.

Some filters are nothing other than taste and odor units and do little to protect your health.

Other Considerations

Currently, there are over 20 major brands of water filters offered on the market. While the most important factor to consider is the degree to which a filter purifies water, there are a few other considerations as well.

1. How does the unit actually perform?

Some filters are nothing other than taste and odor units and do little to protect your health. While an eager salesperson can provide some very convincing "facts," the best way to confirm filter performance is to ask for a "performance data sheet." Also, while most filters may provide lead filtration, the degree to which lead is removed will vary. The performance data sheet will list how well the filter stands up to a variety of the most harmful substances found in drinking water and inform you if it has been certified by your state department of health services and other third-party organizations, such as the highly respected National Sanitation Foundation (NSF).

2. What is the cost of the unit?

How often will you need to replace the filter? While some filter systems have filters that need to be replaced after 250 gallons, others can go for a full 500 gallons before they are in need of replacement. The cost of the replacement filters is another consideration.

3. What is the flow rate of the unit?

Some units, while filtering well, may provide only a "dribble" of purified water at a time. Flow rate is stated in "gallons per minute" and can make quite a difference, particularly for family use.

4. Does the unit have a customer satisfaction guarantee and warranty? All other factors being equal, a guarantee and warranty can make an important difference.

Shower Filtration

It has been estimated that one can be exposed to as much chlorine in an average shower as by drinking 2 litres of chlorinated water. The reason is that with a shower, there is the problem of dermal(skin) absorption, as well as inhalation of the chlorinated vapor. Therefore, it is advised that you invest in a shower filter, as well. Unlike tap filtration systems, there is not much variation in shower filters. Most systems will remove about 85% of the chlorine and need replacing every 6 months. Price ranges from $40-$60. (See Resources for ordering).

As you consider what kind of water filtration system might work best for you, remember that human beings cannot live without water, and pure water provides one of the basic foundations for good health, including the prevention of breast cancer. While requiring a big commitment of resources, pure water will more than pay for itself in the long run if you compare it to the true costs of disease and ill health. Your health is worth it!

CHAPTER TWELVE

Minimizing Exposure to Toxic Chemicals

We have already looked at how agricultural chemicals make their way into our bodies through our diet. By adopting the plant-based diet outlined in this book, and by assuring that you have well-purified water to drink and bathe in, you will be making a significant step toward reducing your intake of cancer-causing agricultural chemicals. What follows are steps you can take to further eliminate toxic chemicals from your home that may be contributing to your risk of breast cancer and other diseases.

PESTICIDES, LAWN, AND GARDENING CHEMICALS
The average American garage contains at least a few chemicals used for killing weeds or fertilizing lawns and other plants. Though it may be difficult to believe at first, most of these chemicals are really not necessary. Today, organic community gardens are springing up all over big cities in America, demonstrating that organic gardening is a viable alternative. In fact, magazines have been launched entirely on the subject of organic gardening, and numerous companies are now marketing non-toxic alternatives for pest control. (See Resources). For your health and the health of your family and pets, this is a wise direction in which to move.

Take a look in your basement, your garage, and your supply closets to see what inventory of gardening chemicals you may be storing. Then seek out a center in your community that assists with proper disposal of such chemicals. Be sure to eliminate all bug sprays, pest strips, ant and rodent poisons, and flea powders and sprays.

Part of eliminating hazardous chemicals from your life is choosing products wisely. Ruth Caplan, author of *Our Earth, Ourselves* offers important advice in this regard. She recommends the following: "For every product in your home, in the supermarket or in a hardware store, think all the way back to where it came from and all the way forward to where it will end up. Pick up a can of bug spray. Think back: Every pesticide manufacturing plant in the U.S. is emitting dangerous materials into the air, land and water. Think forward: Your nearly empty can will end up with millions of others in leaking landfills or polluting incinerators. And don't forget that the actual use of this poison is endangering your health as it settles on your skin and in your lungs. In our intricately connected web of life all these chemicals sooner or later turn up in the air, soil, groundwater, rivers, lakes and oceans as well as in our food and ultimately, our bodies."

Seek out products made by more environmentally responsible companies such as Earth Rite, Planet, and Seventh Generation (See Resources for non-toxic alternative products). These companies manufacture products that are free of harmful chemicals and non-toxic to the environment. Many kitchen cleansers and detergents contain petrochemicals and should be avoided. Seventh Generation, the makers of a line of environmentally safe cleaning and paper products, states that if every household in the United States were to replace just one 32 ounce bottle of petroleum-based glass cleaner with a renewable source, such as their own, 47,000 barrels of oil could be saved — enough to operate an automobile for 49 million miles!

Do not have your home or yard sprayed with pesticides. Do not place "no-pest" pesticide strips in your home, and do not "bomb" your home with pest or flea foggers. These activities will expose you, your family, and any pets to seriously toxic chemicals and sharply increase risk of cancer. (See Resources for makers of alternative pest control products).

COSMETICS

Avoid toxic hair dyes. As mentioned, many commonly used hair dyes contain known human carcinogens. Black and dark brown dyes are particularly risky. Check the label of the product you use and be sure it does not contain phenylenediamine. Seek out alternative hair dyes made from natural pigments (See Resources). Also, many shampoos — even some of those marketed as "natural"— contain unhealthful ingredients, including carcinogens. Avoid shampoos, conditioners and other cosmetics containing Cocamide DEA (an ingredient that can be contaminated with carcinogens), and tooth paste (most major brands) that contains titanium dioxide, saccharin, and FD&C Blue #1, all known carcinogens. Also, avoid fluoride-containing toothpaste. Seek out shampoos, soaps and other cosmetics that contain the least ingredients, and then only those that are proven safe (See Resources).

DRY CLEANERS

We have seen that the popular chemical solvent used in America's 30,000 dry cleaners is a known human carcinogen. *Scientific American* published an article describing how scientists using special equipment can go into a home after dry-cleaned garments are hung in a closet and measure the level of ambient solvent that is outgassing from the clothes. **The residue of this cancer-causing chemical stays in your clothes and may later be absorbed through your skin as you perspire.**

Take a look in your basement, your garage, and your supply closets to see what inventory of gardening chemicals you may be storing.

Today there are a variety of "wet cleaners" opening up around the country. These businesses use safe, non-toxic detergents in place of solvents, and the value and quality of service offered is giving conventional cleaners something to talk about. Seek out such an establishment where you live. (Please see Resources for a wet cleaners directory). Another step you can take is to simply avoid purchasing garments that require special cleaning procedures.

GASOLINE

The state of California requires all gasoline stations to post a hazard warning sign where customers can see it. The sign states clearly that it has been determined that gasoline and its related products are known human carcinogens. In the face of such a warning, Californians and millions of other Americans routinely enter gas stations and pump fuel into their car tank. The process of doing so exposes you to toxic vapor and, in case of accidental spillage, gasoline itself. If you must drive a car, your options are limited in regards to this hazard. Although it costs a bit more per gallon, you may opt for full service and remain in your car while the attendant pumps the gas for you.

It is also common for Americans to keep a spare can of gas in their garage. This hazard may be releasing fumes into the air you breathe in the garage.

HOUSEHOLD CLEANERS AND PAINTS

Much of the household cleaners and spot removers we rely upon today are toxic.* Some, such as many glass cleaners, are petroleum-based. There have been cases where unsuspecting consumers mixed two common household cleaners, and this mix resulted in an explosion! This is a clear indication that such products are dangerous.

Places to Look for Hazardous Chemicals in the Home

Look in your basement, under the kitchen sink, cleaning closet, attic and garage, and yard shed for the following products that may be toxic.

Look for: laundry bleach, disinfectants, ammonia, paints, waterproofers, hair care products, nail polish remover, spot removers, oven cleaners, artist paints, glues, cements, pest sprays, garden chemicals, glass cleaners, photographic chemicals, *pesticides*: pest sprays, no-pest strips, flea powders and sprays, home foggers, lawn chemicals, and yard chemicals.

Examine the products carefully. If the consumer label has any type of warning, or perhaps a skull and cross bones on it, you are likely holding a poison in your hand.

Many household paints are also toxic to humans and animals, and should also be collected by a hazardous waste service. Seek out low-VOC (volatile organic chemicals) paint lines such as Safe-Coat and Allsafe and lines offered by Pratt & Lambert, and Morewear. Non-toxic paints should have a Green Seal on their label.

Many of the chemicals Americans buy are actually quite unnecessary or can be replaced by equally effective non-toxic alternatives. (See Resources).

PAPER PRODUCTS

Avoid all paper products that have been chlorine-bleached. This includes conventional toilet pater, facial tissues, cotton balls, cotton swabs, tampons, tea bags, coffee filters, and paper towels. For all these products there are safer alternatives. Please see Resources for ordering such products.

---

*A comprehensive guide for purchasing safe household products is David Steinman and Samuel Epstein, M.D.'s *The Safe Shopper's Bible* (Macmillan, 1995).

CIGARETTE SMOKE

It is assumed that anyone who is serious about his or her health and about preventing disease will choose not to smoke. However, even the non-smoker is exposed to secondhand smoke in a variety of circumstances. Only recently have consumers learned about the numerous toxic chemicals that are found in cigarettes and their smoke. **While there are over 100 toxic chemicals contained in a single cigarette, a single one, benzo[a]pyrene is known to cause genetic mutations to cells.**[224] Understandably, there are going to be circumstances in which controlling your exposure to second-hand smoke will be difficult. Don't kid yourself by thinking that sitting in a "nonsmoking" section of a restaurant reduces your exposure. Cigarette smoke makes no distinction between smoking and nonsmoking zones, and eventually it will poison all of the air in a restaurant. Fortunately, increasingly strict ordinances in some states are making finding a smoke-free restaurant or nightclub less of a hardship.

CLOTHING

Few people are aware that much of the clothes we wear are grown with the use of enormous quantities of pesticides. This is because cotton, the most common clothing fiber, is treated with more pesticides per acre than almost any crop. In fact, 26 percent of the global pesticide burden comes from cotton production.

Today, an increasing number of companies have realized the importance of offering clothing produced from organic fibers. There are also numerous companies now offering organic cotton diapers and clothing for newborns and toddlers, as well (see Resources). By choosing organic cotton clothing whenever possible, you not only help reduce the payload of pesticides that end up in our air, water and soils, but you also will be assured a source of pesticide-free clothing.

Remove Shoes When Indoors

Make a point of taking your shoes off and leaving them by the door of your home. Most of us unwittingly track a variety of chemicals in to the home on our shoes. As we move about the home, chemical residues (petroleum products from parking lots, pesticides from lawns, etc.) are deposited in carpet fibers and furniture. As an indication of this problem, University of Southern California researchers have found DDT deposits in the carpet fibers of 90 percent of the homes studied.

PLASTICS

It is advisable that you avoid plastics as much as possible, particularly those made from vinyl chlorides (including PVC). Avoid products contained in plastic bottles that have a #3 on the bottom which indicates they are manufactured from PVC. Avoid using plastic food storage containers, plastic wrap, shower curtains (use cotton or other natural fiber), inflatable toys, rainwear, and garden hoses.

CHAPTER THIRTEEN

Avoiding Alcohol

In Chapter 2 alcohol consumption was identified as a risk factor for breast cancer. It has been shown repeatedly that alcohol raises estrogen levels in the body and increases the risk of breast cancer in both premenopausal and postmenopausal women.[225] Researchers at the National Institute of Environmental Health Sciences found that **one drink a day was sufficient to increase breast cancer risk by 10 percent. Two drinks a day increased risk by 20 percent when compared to women who drank no alcohol.**[226] A meta-analysis of 16 studies conducted by researchers at Harvard University suggested that two drinks a day may increase risk by as much as 70 percent when compared to nondrinkers.[227]

Again, there are several reasons alcohol may increase risk. First, as mentioned, alcohol increases estrogen levels.[228] Estro-

Some alcoholic beverages contain known carcinogens, and alcohol also impairs the immune system, which plays a role in keeping cancerous cells in check.

gen is metabolized by way of two paths, one short and the other long. The short path is considered safer because this is how non-cancer-promoting estrogens, such as plant estrogens are transported. The long path is taken by environmental estrogens from industrial chemicals, by estrogens in hormone therapy, and estradiol, the estrogen that seems to be the breast cancer promoter. Alcohol may temporarily inhibit the short route for estrogens to reach receptor sites and, as a consequence, leave receptor sites open for the more dangerous type of estrogen. Additionally, some alcoholic beverages contain known carcinogens, and alcohol also impairs the immune system, which plays a role in keeping cancerous cells in check.[229] Alcohol consumption has also been associated with an increased risk for heart disease.

We have already talked about the serious risk posed by chemical pesticides, and fungicides found in foods, but few people consider the pesticides that end up in the alcoholic beverages they consume. For instance, much of the grape acreage in America and Europe that is used for winemaking is heavily treated with pesticides and fungicides. So, with every glass of nonorganic wine one drinks, they are increasing their body's dose of these toxic chemicals.

Now that you are familiar with a few of the risks associated with alcohol consumption, consider that **the annual per capita consumption of alcoholic beverages by persons over the age of 14 in the U.S. is 14 cases of beer, 12 bottles of wine, and 12 fifths of liquor (distilled spirits).**

Making the Break

Some people can easily make the break from alcohol themselves. Others may need assistance doing so because alcohol has come to play an integral role in their lives. (See Resources for alcohol-related support groups).

The non-alcoholic beverage market has expanded greatly in the last few years. Today, consumers have a choice of organically produced, naturally sparkling wines, naturally flavored mineral waters, nonalcoholic beer, and a variety of other tasty beverages that are intended to replace alcoholic drinks.

CHAPTER FOURTEEN

Exercising for Prevention

In Chapter 7, we learned of the devastating effects of stress on the immune system and the role of stress as a risk factor for breast cancer. This chapter looks at one of the key ways to combat stress while increasing our overall physical well-being: exercise. We feel better with regular exercise because exercise provides an outlet for releasing stress and tension and enables us to control our body weight and increase energy reserves. In the past decade, it has become increasingly clear that regular exercise not only can make one feel good but also offers tremendous benefits in terms of disease prevention and longevity. **Despite this knowledge, about 58 percent of American women lead a sedentary lifestyle.**[230]

Women who lived a sedentary lifestyle were even worse off, having a mortality rate five times higher than the most fit women.

An important study led by Dr. Steven Blair at the world-famous Institute for Aerobics Research involved over 13,000 participants who were monitored over an eight-year period to determine how levels of fitness influenced longevity. Those men who lived the most sedentary lifestyle showed a mortality rate three times higher than that of men who were most physically fit. Interestingly, those **women who lived a sedentary lifestyle were even worse off, having a mortality rate five times higher than the most fit women.**[231]

EXERCISE AND BREAST CANCER RISK

Considering the potency of the protective effect of exercise with regard to breast cancer, it is truly shocking how little attention has been given to this preventive strategy. To date, at least 12 studies have confirmed a powerfully protective effect from regular exercise.[232] The most recent study, the largest of its kind, involved over 25,000 women. Conducted at the University of Tromso in Norway, it found a 52 percent reduction in risk for those women who were the most physically active.[233]

Another study, led by Dr. Leslie Bernstein and colleagues at the USC School of Medicine, showed an even greater benefit. It found that **women who engage in four or more hours of exercise a week during their reproductive years could reduce their risk of breast cancer by up to 60 percent.** It is believed that the protection afforded by exercise during this time comes from the fact that the activity alters menstrual patterns. Specifically, exercise can shorten the luteal phase of the menstrual cycle, when more estrogen is produced, and lengthen the follicular phase, when less estrogen is produced, thereby reducing overall exposure to estrogen.

EXERCISE AND OTHER DISEASES

In addition to reducing risk of breast cancer, a regular exercise program can significantly reduce the risk of numerous other diseases, including heart disease, hypertension, adult-onset diabetes, osteoporosis, and obesity. Again, because hormone replacement therapy is promoted as a means for reducing risk of heart disease and osteoporosis, I will describe how powerful exercise is in reducing risk of these two diseases.

Exercise and Heart Disease

Substantial research has confirmed that regular aerobic exercise is an effective way to help prevent the onset of atherosclerosis, or hardening of the arteries. The protective effect comes from the fact that aerobic exercise alters the balance of fats, which play a role in the development of atherosclerosis, in the blood. Specifically, exercise tends to lower concentrations of triglycerides and LDL cholesterol (the less desirable form of cholesterol) while helping to increase HDL cholesterol (the more desirable form). It has been shown that, when practiced with the dietary and stress-reduction strategies presented in this book, a person can reverse a case of advanced heart disease without drugs or surgery. Imagine that just by becoming aerobically fit you can reduce your chance of heart attack by 50 percent!

Exercise and Osteoporosis

As discussed earlier, osteoporosis is a disease in which bones become progressively porous and frail, leading to increased risk of fracture. For too long this disease has been accepted as an inevitability of age. Furthermore, causes of the disease have been misconstrued, leading many women and men to make ineffective alterations in their lifestyle in hopes that it would reduce their risk. The fact is, as pointed out in Chapter 8, we can do much to help retard if not prevent this disease. Exercise happens to be one of the most potent elements of the preventive package.

The image of bone for most people is a sun-bleached, dried-out, porous carcass in the dessert. This image comes from westerns, or perhaps from actually having seen bones while hiking in the wilderness. The fact is that bone is a living and constantly changing form of tissue. Like muscle, bone is responsive to stimulation and with disuse, begins to shrink. Bones need weight bearing on them to remain stimulated and strong.

In one study it was shown that women who exercised three times weekly for twenty-two months were able to increase their bone mass by over 6 percent, while sedentary women, used as a comparison, lost bone mass.[234]

SUGGESTIONS FOR EXERCISE

When it comes to exercise, what you do is not as important as your doing it regularly. Each individual will gravitate toward one or another form of exercise, whether it be running, speed–walking, stair–climbing, dancing, cycling, swimming, roller-blading, rowing, or cross-country skiing. If you have been fairly sedentary until now, experiment with the different forms of exercise available to you.

The key is regularity. You will benefit most from exercising at least four times a week. Exercising more often is a personal choice. Some people choose to exercise every day because they feel better doing so. This is not necessary. It's best to strive to perform aerobic exercise four days a week for sessions of at least 30 minutes each.

I will not go into the details of how to perform exercises in this text. However, if you are interested, I recommend my book *Whole Health: The Guide to Wellness of Body and Mind*, (Parissound, 1997). *Whole Health* provides over 150 photographs of models performing a wide variety of exercises following correct form, as well as progressive routines beginning at the novice level. The book also contains guidelines for developing your own exercise routines. (See order form at the back of the book).

IS A GYM NECESSARY?

Whether you choose to join a gym depends on what type of exercise you wish to do. Joining a gym may be your best bet, both because of the variety of apparatuses you will have available to you and because you will probably be more likely to follow through with an exercise program if you have spent money on a gym membership.

While some people gravitate toward a single form of exercise, such as running, and don't need access to a gym, I find that many individuals wish to vary their routine, incorporating a variety of movements from time to time. For example, you may start out exercising on the stationary cycle and after some weeks decide to walk or run on a treadmill. Perhaps stair-climbing or rowing is your interest.

Moreover, to gain the full health benefits of exercise, it is essential to incorporate progressive resistance movements that strengthen your muscles. Aerobic conditioning is very important, and aerobic exercise is the type that offers the risk reduction women are looking for. Yet for all the many benefits of exercise (increased coordination, strength, and metabolic rate) you should also include progressive resistance exercises that incorporate free weights or machines. In this case, to really get a good workout, finding an appropriate gym is essential. You want access to the latest equipment and to someone who can be available to spot you or assist you with technique and form. My experience is that people who enjoy exercising alone are the exception.

A blood panel is like a window to the inside of your body and can expose a good deal of what is going on.

Most people find it motivating to exercise with other people who share their interest in health. Being in their presence can be stimulating and can provide encouragement. Finding an exercising companion can help you stay committed to exercise. Knowing you have a friend waiting at the gym for you and expecting you to show up will support you in your desire for health and fitness, and vice versa.

You may wish to employ a progressive resistance program (using weights and machines) following your aerobic workout. Or you may wish to exercise aerobically on different days from your resistance workout. Do what works best for you according to your availability of time and energy.

BEFORE YOU START

Assuming that you have chosen the type of exercise you are going to engage in and the place at which you will be exercising, you need to consider two preliminaries.

First, if you have been fairly inactive, consult your physician. Explain to him or her that you are planning to begin an exercise routine that will include aerobic conditioning and perhaps progressive resistance routines using weights and machines. Knowing this, your physician will be able to determine whether you should limit your activity in any way.

If you are 40 years of age or older, or simply have the inclination, I suggest that your exam include a maximal performance treadmill stress test. Such a test is particularly important if you have a family history of heart disease, know you have elevated cholesterol, smoke cigarettes, or have diabetes. The treadmill test is an effective way to measure your overall level of cardiovascular fitness and determine whether you have a condition that needs special attention.

Regardless of your age, I suggest that you also have a simple blood panel performed. In a ten-minute procedure, your blood is drawn, and a sample is sent to a laboratory for analysis. People can look deceptively healthy on the outside. A blood panel is like a window to the inside of your body and can expose a good deal of what is going on. A panel will reveal such things as your total cholesterol level, HDL level, triglycerides, and glucose. As I have mentioned previously, your cholesterol level is the strongest indicator of your risk for heart disease. Since many women are blindly placed on hormone-replacement therapy in hopes that it will reduce their risk of heart disease, it makes sense to have a clear assessment of what risk already exists.

Finding the Right Club

Once you have received an okay from your physician, you may wish to look around for a health club in your area. Don't rush to join a gym or health club simply because it is convenient. Stop by the club and tell them you are curious about their facility and would like to look around. Some clubs will happily give you a free day pass that you can use to really assess the quality of the place and its equipment. You may want to stop by at different times of the day to see what the atmosphere is like. A gym or health club can be a very different place at 6 P.M. than it is at 6 A.M. simply because of the different numbers and types of people it attracts at different hours.

These days, some clubs offer free personal training for their new members. This is something you may wish to utilize, particularly if you are new to the world of exercise.

Exercise Essentials

Regardless of the types of exercise you perform and where you perform them, it is essential that stretching become a regular part of your routine. Stretching your muscles is an excellent way to prepare them for exercise, increase flexibility and coordination, and facilitate adaptation to regular exercise. Stretching is also an excellent way to loosen up, relieve stressful feelings and muscular tension, increase body awareness, and even enhance circulation. It is an excellent way to relax before going to bed at night, so it needn't be limited to the time that you are exercising. All of these benefits are essential to a preventative lifestyle.

Stretching is not complex or difficult. It requires no equipment, so it can be done anywhere. Since it is noncompetitive, you do it at your own pace, following the signs from your body. There are countless stretches that you can perform, some as basic as those taught in high school physical education classes. The stretches that follow are those that will be most effective for overall conditioning.

How to Stretch

When performing a stretch, ease into the movement rather than bounce or jerk your way through. Too often I see individuals (even professional athletes!) perform ballistic stretches in which they bounce or lurch. These same people often lack flexibility. The reason not to bounce is that ballistic movements put a person head-to-head with a physiological response known as the stretch reflex. This response, a sudden contraction of the muscle being stretched, is a protective reaction that serves to prevent potential tissue damage. The fibers responsible for this response are called the muscle spindles. During a static stretch, where the movement is progressive and controlled, the spindle accompanies the muscle fibers in their elongation. Yet, as soon as it detects movement that could be dangerous, it locks. To avoid this lock-up response, your stretch movements should always be controlled and fluid. At the first sign of tension or resistance, you should stop. Hold the stretch position, usually for 15 to 30 seconds, until the pull has subsided and then continue to move farther into the stretch until the pull is felt again. While stretching, you may become tense and either hold your breath or breathe shallowly. This will counteract your efforts.

Be sure to make a conscious effort to breathe deeply, as this will facilitate your stretching. The distance you move in a stretch could be two inches or two millimeters. What's important is that you focus on the feeling, not on how far you move. Flexibility comes gradually, and the process should never be painful, so don't become frustrated if you can't drop into the splits after a week!

Stretching should be performed before every exercise session, but it can be helpful at other times as well. When stretching before exercise, be sure to warm up your muscles first by performing some light activity such as walking or pedaling a stationary bicycle with no resistance. You can stretch after your exercise session as a way of "warming down" and to reduce the likelihood of soreness from training. Try to get in the habit of stretching whenever you think about it, while talking on the phone or watching television, or even when you're in the bathtub.

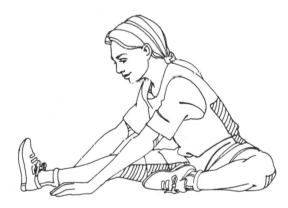

Fig. 1

Hamstring Stretch

Sit on the floor and pull either your left or right leg inward so that the sole of your foot rests next to the inside of the thigh of the extended leg (Fig. 1). Slowly, and from the hip, begin to bend forward in the direction of the foot of the extended leg. As soon as you feel resistance, stop and hold that position for 15 to 30 seconds. Once the resistance has subsided, continue forward until the pulling feeling returns. Hold this position for about 15 seconds. Then stretch the hamstrings of the other leg in the same manner.

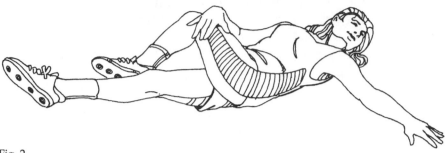

Fig. 2

Lower Back and Hip Stretch

This is one of my favorite stretches for the lower back. Most people find an immediate release of lower back tension when performing this stretch. While lying on your back, bend one knee into a 90-degree angle. Using the hand of your opposite side and placing the palm on the outside of the knee, pull the leg over toward the floor (Fig. 2). Turn your head toward the opposite direction of your bent knee. Relax and hold this position for 15 to 30 seconds. Switch legs and repeat. Don't be concerned if you are unable to touch the floor with your knee. There is no need to force your knee down, either. With time, you will gain an increased range of motion.

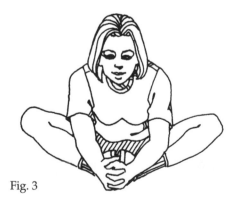

Fig. 3

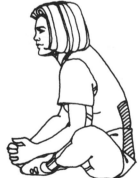

Fig. 3

Groin Stretch

Sitting with the soles of your feet touching each other and your knees facing out to the sides, hold your feet together and move forward from the hips. Pause when you encounter resistance and hold 15 to 30 seconds (Fig. 3). Be sure not to round your back in this movement.

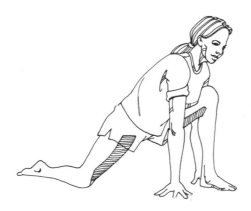

Fig. 4

Hip Flexor Stretch

This stretch will primarily affect the iliopsoas muscles (also known as the hip flexors) located at the front of the hip and may also be felt in the hamstring and groin areas.

From a kneelike position, place your right foot flat on the floor in front of you. Using your hands to support yourself, bend your right knee and extend your left leg behind you. Your right knee should be directly above your right ankle. Rest your left knee on the floor. Allow your hip to move toward the floor for 15 to 30 seconds (Fig. 4). Repeat this movement with your left foot forward. Be sure that the knee of the forward leg is always aligned over the ankle. Flex the buttocks for a better stretch.

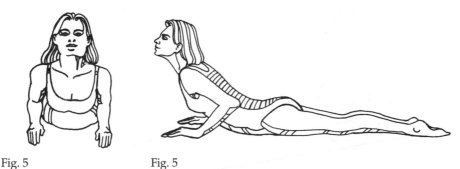

Fig. 5   Fig. 5

Cobra Stretch

Lie on your stomach with your hands shoulder-width apart. Inhale. Gently, push your torso up, exhaling as you go. Hold the stretch for about

15 seconds. Be sure to keep your hips on the floor at all times (Fig. 5). Slowly return to a prone position.

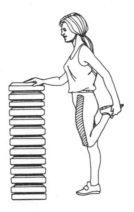

Fig. 6

Thigh Stretch

This movement will stretch the powerful quadricep muscles of the leg. Stand near a wall for stability. Lift either leg behind you, grasp your ankle, and gently pull your leg up behind you. Gradually, bring your heel close to your buttocks and hold this position for 15 to 30 seconds. To enhance the stretch effect, tilt your pelvis forward by contracting your abdominal muscles, then extend the pelvis by contracting your buttocks (Fig. 6). Repeat with the opposite leg.

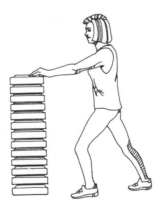

Fig. 7

Calf Stretch

Stand facing a wall or other sturdy structure at arm's length. While keeping one leg straight, place the foot of the other leg in front of you, toes toward the wall (Fig. 7). The rear leg should be kept straight with the heel on the floor. With your forearms against the wall and elbows bent, slowly move forward from the hip. When you feel a pull in the calf of your straight leg, hold the position for 15 to 30 seconds. Do this stretch on both sides.

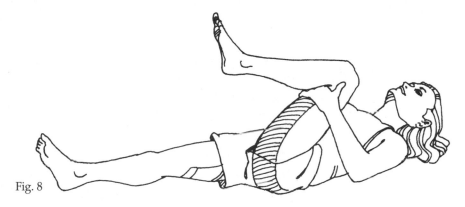

Fig. 8

Low-Back Stretch

Lie flat on your back. With your fingers interlaced under your knee, pull your thigh in toward your chest to increase the stretch. Hold this position for about 15 to 30 seconds (Fig. 8). Switch legs and repeat the movement. This stretch is very relaxing for the lower back and creates an "opening" action in the hips. This movement can also be performed with both legs simultaneously.

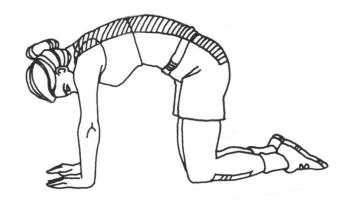

Fig. 9

Cat Stretch

Instinctively, cats perform a stretch similar to this several times a day. Kneel on the floor making sure to keep your knees under your hips and your hands under your shoulders. Inhale. Exhale as you round your back, holding the position for 15 to 30 seconds. This stretch (Fig. 9) can be used interchangeably with the cow stretch.

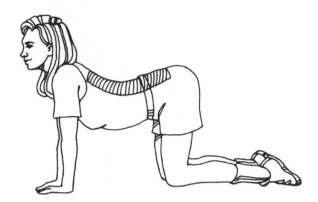

Fig. 10

Cow Stretch

Kneel on the floor, positioning your knees and hands the same as in the cat stretch. Inhale! Exhale as you gently arch your back (Fig. 10).

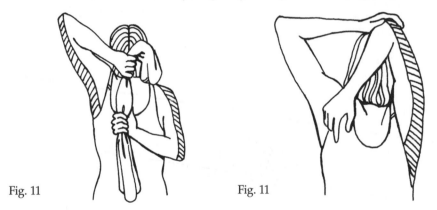

Fig. 11   Fig. 11

Tricep Stretch

As if you were scratching your shoulder, put your right or left arm behind your back. Then, place your opposite hand on top of your elbow. Slowly push the elbow down, until you feel a stretch in the tricep. Hold this stretch for about 15 to 30 seconds. Repeat with the other arm. A variation of this stretch involves using either a broomstick or a towel (Fig. 11).

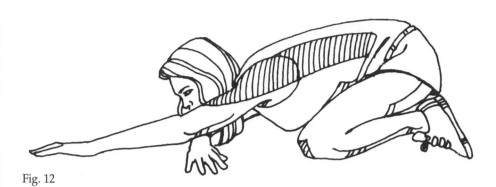

Fig. 12

Back Stretch

This is a great movement for stretching out the latissimus muscles of the back. Kneel on the floor with your forehead resting on your left forearm (Fig. 12). Extend your right arm straight forward. While pressing lightly with your extended palm, pull yourself back slowly. Hold for 15 to 30 seconds. Perform this stretch on both sides.

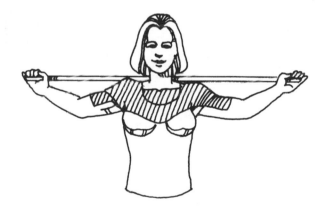

Fig. 13

Chest-Shoulder Stretch

While standing or sitting, grasp a towel or broomstick with an overhand medium to wide grip (Fig. 13). Raise your arms above your body. Then, slowly lower the towel or stick behind your back. To alter the degree of stretch felt in the chest, vary the width of your grip. Hold for about 15 to 30 seconds. A similar stretch can be performed by placing your forearms upright on either side of a doorway and then gently moving forward through the doorway.

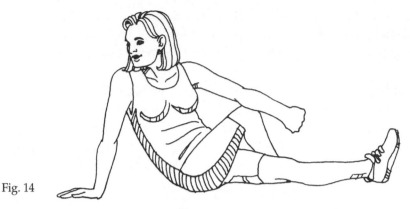

Fig. 14

Twisting Back Stretch

Sit with your back erect and your legs extended in front of you. Bend your right leg and place your right foot on the outside of your left knee. Then place your left elbow against the outside of your right knee. Inhale. Use your right hand to support you as you twist to the right, exhaling as you twist. Slowly return to starting position. Repeat on the opposite side (Fig. 14).

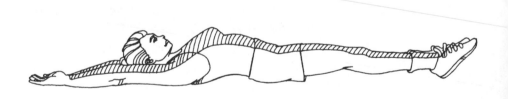

Fig. 15

Full-Body Stretch

This is a wonderful all-body stretch. Lie on your back with your arms extended beyond your head and legs fully extended. Press your lower back against the floor. Reach simultaneously with both your hands and your feet in opposite directions (Fig. 15). Hold this stretch for about 15 seconds and relax. Repeat two to three times.

It's a good idea to stretch before and after exercise. But don't limit yourself to this time! Stretch when you feel tense, when you wake up in the morning, in the bathtub, while watching television, or while talking on the phone. If stretching is not already a part of your life, I know that you will be nicely surprised by the sense of flexibility and general wellness that you will experience.

As you begin to incorporate exercise and stretching into your life on a regular basis, you gain a powerful tool for reducing the risk of breast cancer, heart disease, and other diseases, as well as for managing stress in your life. In the next two chapters, we'll explore additional methods for reducing stress.

AEROBIC EXERCISE

To achieve aerobic fitness, you are aiming to work the heart muscle harder than usual. This is accomplished by exercising at what is known as your *target heart rate* (THR) for at least 20-minutes a minimum four times per week. Your THR is a safe heart rate that allows you to derive the greatest benefits from exercise. Here is how you can calculate your own THR. Subtract your age from 220. This will give you what is called your Predicted Maximum Heart Rate (PMHR) which you should *never* exceed. For best results you should work to raise your heart beats per minute to between 60 percent and 85 percent of your MHR. If you multiply your PMHR times 0.60 you will find your lower guide number. Then, multiply your PMHR by 0.85, and find your upper guide number. Depending on your level of fitness, your THR, expressed in beats per minute, will lie between these two numbers. If you have little or no prior aerobic conditioning, it is advisable that you keep your heart rate closer to 60 percent or less of your PMHR, and work up from there as you become more conditioned. A more active individual should have no problem exercising at 70 percent of their MHR in the beginning. After 10 minutes of exercise you can check your pulse to see if you are exercising at an appropriate rate of intensity and make adjustments accordingly.

Target Heart Rate Example
Age: 35
220 − 35 = 185
MHR = 185
185 x .60 = 111
185 x .85 = 157
Target heart rate falls between 111 and 157

Remember that *the longer you exercise at a time, the more effectively your body will utilize fat stores.* So while normal aerobic conditioning is achieved during training periods of between 20-30 minutes, for enhanced fat loss, it is important to extend the aerobic workout to between 45 and 60 minutes. Although you may feel inclined to increase the intensity of your aerobic exercise, it is best to make increases in both duration and frequency *before* intensity. However, during these extended training periods, it may initially be necessary for you to lower your training heart rate to accommodate the extended duration.

Always remember, aerobic training should not be exhausting. While you should notice an increase in your breathing and pulse rate and a bit of perspiration, you should not feel wiped out. For aerobic exercise to be effective, there must be an adequate supply of oxygen available to the working muscles. When we exercise at too great an intensity, we surpass what is known as the anaerobic threshold. This is the point at which adequate oxygen is no longer available, the body must switch to the anaerobic energy system, and fatty acids are no longer a primary fuel source. As we become more conditioned, our **anaerobic threshold** becomes greater, allowing us to exercise at higher intensities and still remain "aerobic" in effect. While training heart rate is important, a reliable method for checking aerobic intensity is called the "talk test." At any time, you should be able to carry on a conversation with another person without feeling winded.

DETERMINING YOUR PULSE RATE

After exercising for at least five minutes, stop and hold one finger either at your wrist (radial artery) or on the neck to the side of the larynx (carotid artery). Be sure not to apply excessive pressure to the carotid artery because it contains *baroreceptors* that react to such pressure and slow the heart rate. Count the number of beats that occur in a 10-second period. Multiply that number by six to find your heart rate.

Proper Warm-ups

Whatever your target heart rate, you don't want to reach it immediately. It is *imperative* that you warm up before reaching your training heart rate. Warm-ups are really any activity performed at a rate of intensity much lower than when exercising. For example, walking, light jogging in place, and stationary cycling are all effective ways to warm up as long as they are performed for three to five minutes at low intensities. A warm-up period allows the body to acclimate in several ways. First, as the term implies, it increases the temperature of the muscles making them more pliable and less vulnerable to injury. Second, the vascular system adjusts as well, restricting blood flow to the abdominal region and redirecting it to the muscles that are being used and which require a greater oxygen supply. (If you warm up before attempting to stretch, you will find that your flexibility will increase with greater ease).

Proper Cool-downs

Like warming up, cooling down is a crucial part of any aerobic exercise session. After you've exercised, particularly if you've cycled or run, vast quantities of blood are often "pooled" below the waist. If you stop suddenly, there is a risk that circulation to the heart and brain will be compromised, the consequences of which could be severe. Rather than stopping abruptly, progressively reduce the intensity of your exercise over a three– to five–minute cool-down period. This will prevent pooling of blood in the veins allowing for proper circulation throughout the body, and also prevent potential dizziness.

AEROBIC ACTIVITIES

As we have seen, there are many aerobic activities to choose. While some people prefer to perform their aerobic exercise in organized movement classes, many find walking or running preferable because it takes them outside. Further, both of these forms of exercise can be performed just about anytime and anywhere.

Additionally, there are a number of excellent machines and training apparatuses available for aerobic exercise at most health clubs (e.g., stair climber, treadmill, rowing machine, stationary cycle, recumbent cycle, etc).

• Swimming	• Walking	• Running
• Cycling	• Dancing	• Rollerblading/skating
• Jumping rope	• Downhill skiing	• Cross-country skiing

The Walking Program

Probably the simplest form of aerobic activity is walking. Walking is a particularly good choice for those who are significantly overweight (20-30 pounds or more over their desirable weight), those who have led a sedentary life, and anyone who has an orthopedic condition.

While walking does not expend as many calories as other forms of exercise, it can be an effective means of achieving cardiovascular fitness when performed at a brisk rate.

The best way to begin a walking program is to start out walking on flat surfaces such as a bike path or the residential streets in your neighborhood. As the body becomes more conditioned, you can increase the intensity both by increasing the walking pace and by walking on surfaces with a moderate grade. Walking on steep hills is not recommended. Be sure to use the stretching program before and after your walk. Following is a sample walking program that you can adapt to create your own walking program.

15–WEEK WALKING PROGRAM			
Walk (minutes)	Brisk Walk (minutes)	Walk (minutes)	Total (minutes)
WEEK 1 5	1	5	11
WEEK 2 5	2	5	12
WEEK 3 5	5	5	15
WEEK 4 5	8	5	18
WEEK 5 5	10	5	20
WEEK 6 5	12	5	22
WEEK 7 5	15	5	25
WEEK 8 5	17	5	27
WEEK 9 5	20	5	30
WEEK 10 5	22	5	32
WEEK 11 5	25	5	35
WEEK 12 5	27	5	37
WEEK 13 5	30	5	40
WEEK 14 5	32	5	42
WEEK 15 5	35	5	45

Program should be followed three non-consecutive days.

Running Program

Running is also an excellent form of aerobic conditioning that helps develop, strengthen, and condition the muscles you are exercising in the gym. A regular running program offers all the same health benefits of the walking program. Today, it is estimated that 30 million Americans include running in their regular exercise program. *Caution: If you have any type of orthopedic condition (bone or joint problem), running is probably not your best choice for aerobic exercise.*

If you choose to begin running and have no previous experience, I suggest a gradual "break-in" period before you attempt to win any marathons. The best way to start is simply by following the above walking program. As you become more conditioned, instead of brisk walking, you can increase your pace to a jogging and then running pace. Jogging is not running. Think of it as a stage between a brisk walking and running pace. Initially, work from a jog/run/jog period to a full running period between your five–minute warm-up and five–minute cool–down periods. The following table shows is a sample running program you may wish to use as a model in fashioning your own running program.

How to Run

Proper running form not only helps prevent injury and premature exhaustion, but will also make your run more enjoyable. First, make sure to keep your shoulders relaxed at all times. There is a tendency to lift the shoulders and hold them in tensely. When the shoulders are lifted like this, the arms usually end up pinned to the sides of the body. If the arms are relaxed and free, you can move them forward in a pumping motion. This movement will increase momentum and propel you forward with greater ease. Your hands should be loose (not in a fist) and move directly in front of you rather than across your body. Also, avoid landing flat on your feet. It is best to land on the heel of the foot and then roll onto the ball and toe before pressing off again.

Where to Run

It's important to consider the surface on which you run. The sidewalks of most cities are made of concrete, which has very little absorbency. Asphalt, which is used to pave most roads, is slightly better. Some communities have built specific running paths or "par course paths" on the roadsides or through parks. Usually these paths are formed from clay and provide significant shock absorbency. If you have access to such a course, take advantage of it. Another option is to run on a local school or college track. These tracks are usually made of an absorbent material that will significantly reduce impact. Running on a beach is probably the most impact-free alternative, yet you will lose some of the spring gained from running on firmer surfaces. It is best to avoid running on hills. While a moderate incline can be a nice challenge, avoid downhill running because of the stress it places on the shins and lower back.

Running Attire

The most important component of your running attire is shoes. Although the price tag can be as high as some people's car payment, investing in a good pair of running shoes is crucial. Look at it as an investment in your feet. Today, good running shoes have become really high-tech. They are made to cushion and protect your feet while giving ankle support, and they will absorb a lot of the shock encountered when running on hard surfaces. Running shoes are also significantly lighter than tennis shoes and offer greater traction because of larger treaded soles.

The clothes you run in should be loose and allow free movement. If the weather allows, a pair of shorts and a T-shirt are fine. In cooler weather, you may need to dress in layers. Choose clothing made of cotton, fleece-lined cotton, wool, and nylon, as these materials will allow sweat to evaporate. In warmer weather, choose light colors that reflect sunlight. A loose fitting cap is also a good idea. Remember, in warmer temperatures you will perspire considerably more. Be sure to drink plenty of water before and after your run.

The Running Program

The program I have provided is a suggestion of what may work for you. Depending on your physical condition when you start and whether or not you've had running experience, you may need to make some adjustments. That's fine. While I'm suggesting a goal to work toward, there is no reason to push it your first week. If at any time during your running you feel lightheaded, have tension, cramping, or become short of breath, slow to a jog or even a walk. Keep in mind that running, like any form of exercise, should not be painful. Some people are not compatible with running–for whatever reason, they experience discomfort. Others are in their element when they run. Give it a try and see what you think. Remember, as with other aerobic exercises, your goal is moderation. There is no need to race or sprint as doing so can make running more anaerobic. As your running period increases, check your heart rate to be sure you are within your safe range.

Remember to use the stretching program before and after your run. The following table illustrates a progressive 16-week running program that you may wish to model.

15–WEEK RUNNING PROGRAM		
Walk	Jog/Run/Jog	Walk
WEEK 1	5 mins	1 mins	5 mins
WEEK 2	5 mins	3 mins	5 mins
WEEK 3	5 mins	5 mins	5 mins
WEEK 4	5 mins	7 mins	5 mins
WEEK 5	5 mins	10 mins	5 mins
WEEK 6	5 mins	12 mins	5 mins
WEEK 7	5 mins	15 mins	5 mins
WEEK 8	5 mins	17 mins	5 mins
WEEK 9	5 mins	20 mins	5 mins
WEEK 10	5 mins	22 mins	5 mins
WEEK 11	5 mins	25 mins	5 mins
WEEK 12	5 mins	27 mins	5 mins
WEEK 13	5 mins	30 mins	5 mins
WEEK 14	5 mins	32 mins	5 mins
WEEK 15	5 mins	35 mins	5 mins

Program should be followed three non-consecutive days.

CHAPTER FIFTEEN

Learning to Relax

This chapter is about learning to relax, a key ingredient in minimizing the negative effects of stress on your health, and thereby decreasing your risk for breast cancer. Not only is relaxation an effective means for diffusing feelings of anxiety and tension, numerous studies have demonstrated that, after periods of relaxation, levels of the stress hormones (cortisol and adrenaline) that can impair immune function drop significantly. Studies have also shown that after periods of deep relaxation, T-cell counts that were previously depressed through high stress became elevated to more normal levels. The more one relaxes, the more one's T-cell count rises. The more adept one is at maintaining a relaxed state the more improvement is seen in NK cell activity. **In one study, in which residents of a retirement community were taught relaxation exercises, NK cell activity improved by as much as 30 percent.**

The more we practice relaxation exercises, the less likely that muscular tension and stress will accumulate within our body.

Relaxation is something we can use both when we are in a stressful situation and as a regular practice — a form of preventive maintenance.

Some people believe that they are very relaxed throughout the day. Yet even those who work in the most hassle-free, low-stress environments experience physical and emotional stresses of which they are not aware. You may or may not be very relaxed at this moment as you read these words. Check your shoulders. Are they tight and retracted? Try letting your shoulders drop, releasing them as though they were very heavy. Were you previously holding them tightly? Now check your jaw. Is it clenched? Are you grinding your teeth? Allow your jaw to become heavy, release it, and let it drop. Are your toes clenched in your shoes? Many of us hold parts of our body in tight and clenched positions, even in relaxed situations. Doing this uses energy. Yet we have been doing it so long that we are not even aware of it. After using the following relaxation techniques, you will become much more aware of the subtle ways in which we create physical tension. With practice, you will be able to bring your body easily into a deeply relaxed state, regardless of the activity or situation.

Since a state of relaxation is the antithesis of a state of physical stress, it is clear how important relaxation exercises can be, during times of stress and even when we are more relaxed, as a means of further inoculating ourselves against a stressful reaction in the first place. The more we practice relaxation exercises, the less likely that muscular tension and stress will accumulate within our body.

Deep breathing is an instant antidote to feelings of stress. It releases feelings of tension in the muscles and has a wonderful calming effect on the emotions.

Even during a moderately stressful response, our breathing is likely to become quick and shallow. In full-blown stress reactions, our breathing may become excessively rapid and shallow. This is called hyperventilation. Few of us think about our breath throughout the day. Even when we are not exposed to a stressor, our breathing is likely to be shallow. Shallow breathing expels less carbon dioxide from the lungs and takes in less life-supporting oxygen to the lungs and the rest of the body. When we breathe deeply, we can bring in up to seven times more oxygen than with unconsciously shallow breathing.

ABDOMINAL BREATHING

Most of us are chest breathers. When we breathe with our chest, our abdomen moves in when we inhale and out when we exhale. However, abdominal breathing allows us to utilize the full capacity of our lungs. In abdominal breathing, the abdomen expands as we inhale and pulls in as we exhale. This type of breathing results in more room for the lungs to expand and contract, and, thus, more fresh oxygen intake and more carbon dioxide release.

Take a moment right now to learn the difference between abdominal and chest breathing. Sit up straight in a chair or on the edge of a bed. Place one hand on your abdomen area. Slowly inhale deeply, allowing your abdominal muscles to expand. Then exhale fully, pulling the abdominal muscles in tightly. You will notice that the tighter you pull in your abdominal muscles, the more air will be forced out of your lungs. Take another couple of deep breaths and practice making your abdominal muscles expand outward on the inhalation and contract inward on the exhalation.

Deep abdominal breathing is something you can practice each day. Begin your mornings with two or three minutes of deep abdominal breathing. You will feel refreshed and energized. At times when you feel yourself becoming stressed, you can quickly diffuse the feelings and return to a state of deep calm simply by performing several deep abdominal breaths in succession.

THE TENSION-RELEASE METHOD

The Tension-Release Method is another effective way to teach your body to relax. By experiencing your muscles in a high state of tension, you will better be able to recognize when your muscles "slip" into such a state. By tensing and then relaxing your muscles, you will enable them to relax much more deeply than by simply trying to relax mentally. This exercise involves moving through the entire musculature of the body, tensing and then relaxing small groups of muscles, one at a time.

Choose a time when you will be free from interruption. Lie down on a bed or the floor and close your eyes. Begin by taking four deep breaths. Inhale deeply through your nose, and exhale completely through your mouth. Place your arms at your sides, with your palms facing up and legs extended fully. You will progressively tense every muscle in your body, either one at a time or in pairs.

You may prefer to begin at your head and work down to your feet or the reverse. It makes no difference. For example, begin at the head by raising your eyebrows as high as possible, and furrowing your forehead. Hold this tensed position for five seconds, and then let go. Feel the muscles of your upper face relaxing. Move to your nose and eyes. Close both eye lids tightly while wrinkling your nose, hold them for five seconds, then release them. Moving to your mouth, make a broad and exaggerated smile, holding it for five seconds and releasing. Feel your face relaxing more deeply. Now move to your neck. Slowly pull your head up and bring your chin toward your chest, hold for five seconds, and relax. Now move your head backwards, feeling your neck crease. Hold and relax. Now raise your shoulders up toward your ears, tensing them for five seconds, and releasing. Moving to your upper arms, lock your elbows and tighten the tricep muscles of the back of your arms for five seconds and release them. Then curl your lower arm up and squeeze the bicep muscles tightly for five seconds and release. Now make a fist with each hand and squeeze the fists tightly for five seconds and release. Move to your stomach area and tighten your abdominal muscles for five seconds and release. Moving to your upper legs, lock your knees to tightly tense your thigh muscles for five seconds. To tense the lower leg muscles, aim your toes up toward you, with your heel out. Then push your toes away, pulling your heel in. Hold both of these positions for five seconds and relax them.

In one final contraction, squeeze all of the muscles you have covered simultaneously for five seconds, and then release them. Your body should feel thoroughly relaxed at this point. A very helpful addition is to softly instruct yourself with the word relax each time you release a muscle that has been tensed. This will not only aid in your relaxation session, but you will begin to anchor the word relax with the feeling of a fully relaxed muscle. Then, in anxiety-provoking situations, you can simply scan your body to find areas that are tense and tell yourself to relax. This is an effective tool for getting in touch with tension.

With practice, you will become very sensitized to what your muscles feel like when they are tense, and what they should feel like in a relaxed state. At that point, you will no longer need to move through this entire tension-release process. Instead, you will simply be able to command yourself to relax and feel the deeply relaxed state in your muscles and body. Throughout the day you can do this Tension-Release Method on specific areas that you notice becoming tense. Perhaps it's your shoulders when you are seated at your office desk or your hands gripping the steering wheel of your car. You can perform this relaxation technique as a way of overcoming mild insomnia and assuring deep sleep. You can also use it before taking an exam or making a public presentation, or before an important interview.

Both deep abdominal breathing and the Tension-Release Method can serve you well as you begin to relax and let go of the stress in your life. By dealing with stress proactively rather than letting it build up and control you, you act once again to reduce your risk for breast cancer.

CHAPTER SIXTEEN

Meditation for Prevention

We have looked at how exercise and other forms of relaxation can help reduce the stress that exposes us to an increased risk of breast cancer. In this chapter, we will explore one of the most ancient and time-tested antidotes to stress: meditation.

Every day we are exposed to countless people, events, sounds, thoughts, sensations, feelings, memories, and images. Even though we may go home at the end of the day and be in an environment with fewer people, events, and congestion, many of us continue to maintain a significant amount of mental traffic right up to the moment we fall asleep. The information can flow like a tap, flooding our minds with too much clutter. We may think something like, "It's getting late, better get to sleep . . . did I lock the door? . . .

Many people erroneously believed that meditation was only associated with religion, finding God, becoming a cultist, or "becoming one with the universe."

dinner was good . . . what's on the agenda for tomorrow . . . wow, I forgot to write that paper . . . oh, that TV show is on, I don't want to miss it . . . where is that paper I was reading? Whose dog is that barking? . . . wish I had a dog." If you have a family that you are responsible for, your mental traffic is only compounded.

Meditation is a path away from this bombardment of internal and external stimuli; it is a mental retreat to a place of peace and quiet where the mind becomes calm. Meditation takes us out of the past and the future and brings us into the present. It is calming, yet at the same time heightens our awareness. It develops skill in concentration and focus, which in turn assist us in problem solving and successfully reaching goals.

Up until the early 1970s, meditation had largely been ignored as a means of enhancing one's health. Many people erroneously believed that meditation was only associated with religion, finding God, becoming a cultist, or "becoming one with the universe." Meditation can be and is most commonly practiced independently of any religious affiliation, philosophy, or belief.

Those who meditate regularly have demonstrated the ability not only to alleviate stressful feelings and achieve a deep state of relaxation, but also to reduce their blood pressure, heart rate, rate of respiration, and oxygen consumption. Long-term meditators have also been found to have lower levels of the stress hormones cortisol and adrenaline. Some researchers say that because of these changes, long-term meditators can effectively slow the rate at which they age.

Suffice it to say that as we develop our ability to meditate, to become focused and totally present, we can enable profound changes to occur within our bodies, changes that ultimately will allow us to achieve and maintain a greater level of health. Some ancient meditation techniques have proven to allow physiological changes to occur that seem almost miraculous. For example, in his excellent book *Timeless Healing*, Dr. Herbert Benson, a renowned Harvard stress researcher, tells of his experience meeting with the Buddhist Tibetan monks in India's Himalayan mountains. There, Dr. Benson and his researchers witnessed monks who, by focusing their mind with crystal-clear intention, could, in temperatures of 40 degrees Fahrenheit, dry wet, cold towels placed over their naked bodies.

A study published in the journal *Hypertension* and led by researcher Robert Sneider, M.D., showed that **regular meditation can have the same blood-pressure-lowering effect as medications currently used by hypertensives.**

Other studies are demonstrating that regular meditation not only plays an important role in reducing stress but also that it may be effective in reducing cholesterol levels, chronic pain, and sleep disturbances. In one study, five participants reduced their serum cholesterol by between 4 percent and 9 percent, and three by as much as 35 percent. In another study, meditators showed 80 percent fewer cases of heart disease and 50 percent fewer cases of cancer than those who did not meditate regularly. The landmark Lifestyle Heart Trial, conducted by Dean Ornish, M.D., and his associates, demonstrated for the first time that atherosclerosis can be reversed through comprehensive lifestyle changes. An essential component of the stress-reduction portion of this program was regular meditation.

The fact that meditation can play such a powerful role in controlling cholesterol levels is obviously important in terms of risk of heart disease. It is also important to note the study documenting reduced risk of cancer. When we react to stressful situations negatively, this does more than make us feel bad. Indeed, it takes a serious toll on all the systems of the body, not the least of which is the immune system. When the functions of our immune system are compromised, we not only are more vulnerable to opportunistic diseases but also increase our risk of developing diseases such as cancer. The immune system plays a role in protecting us from cancer by using specialized cells called NK cells. NK cells patrol the body looking for tumor cells and disposing of them before they can become unmanageable.

In another study, meditators showed 80 percent fewer cases of heart disease and 50 percent fewer cases of cancer than those who did not meditate regularly.

Like other forms of deep relaxation, meditation allows the body to return to homeostasis. In this state, all of the interrelated systems, the immune system in particular, can function at their optimal level.

Meditation is really a matter of reaching a state of mindfulness. Jon Kabat-Zinn, Ph.D., founder of the Stress Reduction Clinic at the University of Massachusetts Medical Center, describes this state as "paying attention in a particular way: on purpose, in the present moment, and nonjudgmentally. This kind of attention nurtures greater awareness, clarity, and acceptance of present-moment reality. It wakes us up to the fact that our lives unfold only in moments. If we are not fully present for many of those moments, we may not only miss what is most valuable in our lives, but also fail to realize the richness and the depth of our possibilities for growth and transformation."

Many of us are living far from the present. We spend our time and energy in the past and the future, being guided by a barrage of irrational thoughts, many at an unconscious level. In meditation, we can climb out of this mental traffic — the dreams, worries, thoughts, and fantasies of every day — and become a quiet observer in a place of "pure awareness."

With practice, the awareness of the thoughts, feelings, and sensations you gain through your meditation will spill over into times when you are not meditating. This increased awareness or presence will help prevent irrational thoughts and debilitating reactions to stressors you may encounter and allow you to experience more enjoyment each minute of each day.

HOW TO MEDITATE

These simple guidelines can help you experience successful meditation sessions.

1. Meditate at least an hour after eating, because digestion will prevent you from being totally alert.

2. Choose a place that is quiet and where you are unlikely to be disturbed by a phone ringing or other interruptions.

3. Find a comfortable position that you can maintain for at least 20 minutes. A traditional position involves sitting on your knees with your big toes touching and buttocks resting on your feet. For some, sitting cross-legged, either on the floor or on a cushion, is most comfortable. Others sit with their legs extended straight before them and their back supported, while others choose to lie down or sit in a straight-back chair. Do whatever is most comfortable for you.

There are two popular ways to meditate: one involves counting breaths, and the other involves repeating what is known as a mantra. Experiment with both to see which is most effective for you.

Breath-Counting Meditation

In breath-counting meditation, you breathe through your nose at all times. After finding yourself in a comfortable position, take a deep breath using the abdominal breathing style discussed earlier. As you exhale, say to yourself, "One." With each exhalation repeat to yourself, "One." An alternative is to continue counting with each exhalation until you reach "Four" and then return to "One."

Some people prefer counting to "one" because it takes their focus off of reaching a goal, even if that goal is simply to reach four, and makes it easier for them to stay in the present moment.

Mantra Meditation

In mantra (*man* means "to think," and *tra* means "to liberate") meditation, you will be repeating a name or syllable throughout the meditation session. Common mantras used in the Eastern tradition are *om*, which means "I am," *so-ham*, which means "I am he," and *sa-ham*, which means "I am she." Yet a mantra does not necessarily need to have meaning to anyone other than yourself. It can be simply a sound or two syllables of your own choosing. You can also choose words such as *calm* or *relaxed* as your mantra.

Once you have chosen a mantra, begin your session by chanting the mantra aloud. After about five minutes, you may find yourself feeling centered, and you can then chant silently.

With either breath counting or mantra chanting, the key to your meditative session is to remain calm and relaxed and not judge what is happening. Slow and deepen your breath and remain completely passive. If your mind begins to drift, gently bring the focus back to your breath, observing your inhalation and exhalation. With practice, you will find it easier and easier to remain focused and free of intruding thoughts. However, even advanced meditators become distracted by thoughts and consider the process of noticing the phenomenon and returning to breath simply part of the practice. Do not become concerned over whether or not you are meditating properly. Do not judge your meditation — just experience the calm and relaxed state it brings. If you find yourself judging, simply observe that, too, and then let it go, coming back to the process.

After you have been meditating for some time and you feel comfortable with the process, you may find that you experience a voice. Some say that they hear their "inner voice" or their "higher self." You may choose to ask a question, or you may not. Perhaps you will hear words of wisdom or answers to questions you have. Some people say that this inner dialogue comes naturally to them and is enlightening; others don't experience it at all. Whatever you experience is right for you.

How Often to Meditate

Meditation is best practiced as often as possible, with your goal being sessions of at least 20 minutes each day of the week. You can certainly meditate longer than 20 minutes if you wish, but if 20 minutes is not possible, it's best to meditate every day, even if just for 10-minute sessions. Initially, it may take you a while to become completely relaxed and clear your mind of the mental chatter. However, as you become more experienced, you will attain this calm state more quickly. Ideally, you should set aside a specific time each day to devote to meditation. Perhaps it will be early in the morning before work or school, in the middle of the day at your lunch hour, or just after you arrive home in the evening. At home, make a point of meditating in the same place so there won't be new distractions and adjustments to make with each meditation session.

Mini-Meditations

As pointed out, the essence of meditation is for one to become present, to become aware, to get out of the past and future and be with the moment at hand. Ideally, as described, you find a place and a time to meditate that is most conducive for your practice. However, know that even when you have little time and less than ideal surroundings, you can still practice what I call mini-meditations. This is nothing other than employing some of the same strategies as described earlier but in an ultra-brief setting. Thich Naht Han describes in his book *Peace Is Every Step* that one can use a stop sign as a reminder not only to stop one's car but also to "stop" one's mind. When you see a stop sign, that's your signal to really become present. Stop the car, breathe deeply a few times, let go of any stress that you are holding in your body, and then move on. Depending on the intersection, whether it is busy or not, you may find that you can wait for a few moments safely and comfortably. Stopping your car at the corner of 42nd and Broadway in New York City, however, will definitely not be conducive to waiting a few moments before moving on.

Some other opportunities for relaxing your body and mind and increasing your awareness of the influence you have over your physical and emotional states are available in biofeedback training, yoga, and tai chi, which is actually, a form of moving meditation.

Remember, whatever you can do to reduce stress in your life will help you reduce your risk for breast cancer.

CHAPTER SEVENTEEN

The Seven Steps in Review

The following seven steps are recommended for reducing your risk of breast cancer and improving your health in general. They summarize and highlight the ideas covered in the earlier chapters. Remember, this is not a part-time or "when you feel like it" plan. This is a comprehensive lifestyle program that is intended to be followed full-time. The more of these steps you adopt in your lifestyle, the more you reduce your risk for breast cancer and a host of other diseases and the better your overall health will be.

Step One: Follow the Revised American Diet™

The standard American diet poses considerable risk to your health. By following a plant-based diet, you significantly lower your intake of cholesterol and saturated fat that contribute to the clogging of arteries and you sharply reduce your intake of toxic chemicals, such as pesticides, that concentrate in the fat of animals. Additionally, you will eliminate your exposure to the residues of powerful hormones used to raise farm animals, as well as other products unsuitable for human consumption but typically found in meats and dairy products.

A health-supporting diet contains an abundance of vegetables, fruits, whole grains, and legumes. It may also contain a minimum of raw nuts and seeds for those who enjoy them and do not have difficulty digesting them and are not struggling with a weight problem.

The Revised American Diet™ avoids rancid, hydrogenated, and fried oils. You would be prudent to avoid French fried potatoes and onion rings as well, even though they are made from plants. This also means avoiding pretty much any conventional oils sold in markets today. The exception is cold-pressed, organic, extra virgin olive oil that is sold in opaque glass containers that protect it from light. In addition, remember to avoid refined sugars and grains.

Review Chapters 19-22 for more details on overcoming the Standard American Diet and replacing it with the healthful Revised American Diet.™

Step Two: Choose Organically Grown Foods

Chapters 6 and 10 described some of the hazards associated with consuming pesticide-tainted foods, and Chapter 10 pointed out the importance of choosing organic alternatives whenever possible. The problem of pesticide contamination is far worse than most of us can begin to imagine. Every time that you have a choice, choose organic over conventional fruits, grains, vegetables, herbs, and spices. Yes, the cost is still a bit higher than that of conventional foods, but your health is well worth it! Also, pay attention to the ingredients in packaged foods. Many of the popular snack foods that are turning up in natural foods markets are sweetened with grape juice instead of refined white sugar. While at first this seems safer for one's health, the reality is that grapes are one of the most heavily treated fruits on earth. They receive an enormous quantity and variety of pesticides. When you do buy packaged foods, look for those that have been made from organic ingredients.

Step Three: Consume Only Purified Water

Chapter 6 looked at the current problems of drinking water in America. As described in Chapter 11, the simplest and most efficient strategy to ensure that you obtain purified water is to purchase a point-of-use filtration system for your sinks, ice maker, and even showerheads. Guidelines for making such purchases are also listed in Chapter 11. Keep in mind that when you eat out, the restaurants will in most cases be serving you the same highly chlorinated tap water laden with a host of other contaminants. In this case, choose glass bottled water instead. Some restaurants are now offering filtered water, but don't assume that this is the case. Avoid plastic jugs of water sold at the supermarket. There is evidence that the plastics may leach endocrine-disrupting chemicals and other contaminants into the water at warmer temperatures. Furthermore, the earth simply cannot contend with the loads of plastic containers that are inundating our landfills.

Step Four: Minimize Your Exposure to Toxic Chemicals

Take a good look around your home. You may be surprised by the number of toxic chemicals you harbor under your kitchen sink and in the bathroom, the basement, and the garage. Review the common sources of household toxic chemicals covered in this section.

Today there are safe alternatives for most any household need. Seek them out after safely disposing of those you find around your house. If you are using chlorine-based bleach in your laundry, you are dumping a highly toxic and carcinogenic product into the water with every load and exposing yourself to the fumes at the same time. Seek out alternative, environmentally safe laundry whiteners.

Consider that if every household in America were to replace the 32-ounce bottle of chlorine-based bleach (the stuff most people buy) with one bottle of non-chlorine bleach (See Resources), we could prevent 4.5 million pounds of cancer-causing chlorine from entering our environment annually. Imagine if we kept on using non-chlorine bleach. The potential is great!

Be mindful of the fact that golf courses are a major hazard when it comes to pesticide exposure. In fact, it has been estimated that maintaining the pristine appearance of golf courses may use up to four times more pesticide per acre than farmers do on food crops . . . and a number of these chemicals are endocrine disruptors.[235] The authors of *Our Stolen Future* aptly advise that, if you are a golfer, you may wish to ask the groundskeepers when they apply pesticides, so you can plan to play at different times. Also, be sure to keep your hands away from your mouth while on the course, and wash them thoroughly when leaving the course.

Finally, avoid plastic wrap and plastic water bottles, jugs, and storage containers, and avoid canned foods. Not only are the cans lined with plastic, which can leach into the food, but also, canned foods are nutritionally inferior to fresh foods.[236] Every time that you have a choice, purchase products in glass instead of plastic. This includes cosmetics.

Step Five: Avoid Alcohol

We are very casual about social drinking in the U.S., and it is easy to lose touch with the amount of alcohol we consume. As previously mentioned, the annual per capita consumption of alcoholic beverages by persons over the age of 14 in the U.S. is 14 cases of beer, 12 bottles of wine, and 12 fifths of liquor (distilled spirits). For the reasons indicated earlier, alcohol consumption poses a risk on a number of fronts. The best approach is to quit "cold turkey." Another option is to seek out the assistance provided by such support groups as Alcoholics Anonymous. If you are a drinker, begin stocking your home with and requesting at bars, mineral water, non-alcoholic wines, sparkling cider, and other replacement drinks.

Whether you make the break from alcohol by yourself or with assistance, you will undoubtedly notice a refreshing change in the way your body and mind feels. Depending on how much alcohol you consume, you may also notice additional weight loss once you eliminate alcohol from your life.

Step Six: Exercise Regularly, and Reduce Stress

Chapter 14 outlined the essential role of exercise in helping you cope with stress. It also provided an introductory stretching program. It is entirely your choice what exercise you will do. The idea is to perform some sort of activity that is vigorous and will elevate your heart rate. It might be running or exercising on a stationary bicycle. Your best bet is to join a well-equipped athletic club where you will have access to the greatest variety of current equipment. This way you will be free to choose from any number of exercises and to fashion different routines according to your needs. You may also wish to hire a personal trainer initially as a form of inspiration and to be sure that you become familiar with proper form and technique in exercising. Other forms of stress reduction are also important, and include abdominal breathing and the Tension-Release Method described in Chapter 15.

Seek out products made by more environmentally responsible companies such as Earth Rite, Planet, and Seventh Generation.

Step Seven: Meditate

As Chapter 16 described, this powerful form of stress reduction has been shown to benefit health in numerous important ways, including lowering blood pressure, cholesterol levels, and resting heart rate. Regular meditation allows your body and all of its interdependent systems, not the least of which is the immune system, to function at their optimal levels. The wonderful thing about meditation is that it costs nothing — there are no membership dues for a facility, and you can practice it virtually anywhere, anytime. Other forms of stress reduction that you may wish to explore include various types of tai chi and yoga.

Follow the Seven Steps to Breast Cancer Prevention

Step One: Follow the Revised American Diet™
Step Two: Choose organically grown foods
Step Three: Consume only purified water
Step Four: Minimize your exposure to toxic chemicals
Step Five: Avoid alcohol
Step Six: Exercise regularly, and reduce stress
Step Seven: Meditate

By integrating these seven basic steps into your daily life, you are empowering yourself and reducing your risk of breast cancer as well as a host of other debilitating conditions and diseases. The increased vitality and well-being you'll experience will be your daily reward. I wish you health and vitality as you put these steps into practice.

CHAPTER EIGHTEEN

Protecting the Next Generation

In the beginning of this book, I listed the scientifically accepted risk factors for breast cancer. Some of these factors are immutable, such as sex, race, or family history. A number of other risk factors simply cannot be addressed for a large number of women because they deal with lifestyle choices occurring very early in life. With the knowledge of these risk factors, however, we can now do much to reduce the number of risk factors the next generation will face.

Cancer is currently the leading cause of disease-related death in children between the ages of 1 and 14.[237] Some 40 percent of American children ages 5 to 8 are obese, or have elevated cholesterol or high blood pressure. Children younger than 10 have been found to already have plaque developing in their arteries. Further, each year, about 1,000 teenagers will suffer a stroke caused by symptoms of a high-fat diet, high blood pressure and atherosclerosis. When we look at the types and quantities of foods being consumed by children today, such cases of disease are not surprising.

Currently in America we have a population of girls as young as seven having their periods and developing breasts.

It's not just the food children eat at home either. The average American school menu is a nutritional disaster composed of surplus animal products forced upon schools by farm-subsidy programs.

We have a unique opportunity to reduce not only the risk of breast cancer, but to dramatically improve the general health of the next generation of women (and men).

For example, we know that early menarche is a risk factor for breast cancer because it exposes females to as many as five years more of heightened estrogen levels, and we also know that a high-fat diet and sedentary lifestyle are contributing factors for early menarche. Therefore, we should strive to raise children on the preventive diet outlined in Part Two of this book — a diet that is based on plant foods and composed of whole grains, legumes, leafy greens, vegetables, and fruits. Doing so will not only reduce the overall fat intake for your children but also instill healthy eating habits early in their life that are likely to last a lifetime, thereby reducing their risk of breast cancer as well as other various cancers, heart disease, hypertension, stroke, obesity, osteoporosis, and diabetes. For the same reason, encouraging exercise is also very important as a controllable risk factor. There is more that we can do, however, and this section is devoted to guidelines for maximally reducing risk in the next generation.

PROTECTING YOUR CHILD BEFORE BIRTH

Since most toxic chemicals can cross the placental barrier, a pregnant mother risks exposing her developing fetus to the same chemicals with which she comes in contact. Evidence is mounting that prenatal exposure to a variety of pesticides and other toxic chemicals can have a devastating effect on the future health of a child.[238]

In Chapter 5 we looked closely at the dangers of endocrine–disrupting chemicals. The risk of exposure to such chemicals for adults is serious enough, but it is a powerfully unique risk for the developing fetus. Peter de Fur, a member of the Board of Environmental Sciences and Toxicology for the National Research Council / National Academy of Sciences cautions that "during certain periods of fetal development the [human] is exquisitely sensitive. Only a few cells form the core for [a] new organ . . . If just one or a handful of those cells have a chemical stimulus that alters their developmental path, then the effect is magnified over time in a replication of error," potentially resulting in damage to the reproductive, nervous, and immune systems, and future endometriosis, testicular cancer, attention deficit disorder (ADD), lowered T-cell production, and breast cancer.[239]

What we are seeing today is not far from these projected manifestations. Worldwide sperm counts have dropped 50 percent since 1940*, prostate cancer in men occurs at a rate equal to breast cancer in women, testicular cancer is on the rise, hypospadias, a form of hermaphroditism in which the urethra is exposed on the underside of the penis has doubled since 1968 according to the Center for Disease Control, ectopic pregnancies are up 400% since 1970, and cryptorchidism, in which the testicles do not descend is rising sharply. In wildlife we are seeing the very same conditions and more, such as facial tumors and lack of scales in some fish, hermaphroditic genitalia, club feet and missing eyes, and nesting behavior in male birds. While we can not say for sure that exposure to endocrine-disrupting chemicals is at the root of this health crises, there is strong evidence indicating that it is. For example, many of these conditions can be created in animals simply by altering hormone exposure during different stages of pregnancy.

It has been theorized that if a human fetus is exposed to endocrine-disrupting chemicals, like the animals have been in experiments, a "saturation" of hormonally-responsive tissue may occur that could manifest later in life as tissues with excessive hormone receptors that may ultimately heighten risk of the hormone-dependent cancers such as breast and prostate cancer. Clearly, we need to do everything in our power to protect the next generation from such an assault.

Because it is the most concentrated source of bioaccumulated toxic chemicals (including endocrine-disrupting chemicals), one of the most important things a mother can do is avoid dietary animal fat. Following the Revised American Diet will make this goal easy to achieve.

GROWING UP TOO FAST CAN HAVE GRAVE CONSEQUENCES

As we have seen in earlier chapters, breast cancer is a hormone-dependent cancer. It develops in the presence of the hormone estrogen. As indicated in Chapter 2, of all the scientifically accepted risk factors for breast cancer, cumulative lifetime exposure to estrogen stands out as paramount.

We also know that diet plays a significant role in breast cancer risk — quite possibly the most significant controllable factor to consider. One of the primary reasons is that diet alters the body's production of sex hormones.

This dietary influence on hormones can begin very early in life and thereby set the stage for cancer later in life. Here's how.

When a woman consumes a high-fat diet, her body produces more estrogen. In a pubescent girl, this rise in estrogen can instigate menstruation at an earlier age than if the dietary fat intake had been more moderate. Additionally, when estrogen levels are increased and a high-fat diet containing little fiber is followed, the body's ability to excrete excess estrogens before they are reabsorbed is lessened, heightening risk further. As noted in Chapter 2, early menses is a risk factor for breast cancer.

Early Menses

As stated in Part One, at the turn of the century, the average age at which a woman began menstruating was 17.5 years of age. Today, the average age is 12.5. As mentioned earlier, large numbers of girls in the U.S. are showing signs of puberty by age 7, and in some cases by age 3.[240] With this drop in age has come a concomitant rise in the incidence of numerous diseases including breast, uterine, and ovarian cancer.

We say that menses is a rite of passage, a much-celebrated time when a girl enters womanhood. While such a change may indicate that a girl's body is becoming capable of giving birth, a 12-year-old is hardly physically, let alone emotionally, prepared to become a mother or to contend with the attention a developing woman may receive from males. Currently in America we have a population of girls as young as seven having their periods and developing breasts. Not only is this problem clearly playing a part in the epidemic rates of breast cancer, but it may well play a part in the incredible number of unwanted pregnancies in America each year.

It has been estimated that breast cancer risk is increased 4.2 times in women who reach menarche before age 13. The good news is that researchers have estimated that the risk of breast cancer can be reduced by 10 percent to 20 percent for each year that menarche is delayed.[241]

Two factors may be playing a role here: diet and exposure to toxic chemicals, including pesticides. In one study, published in *New Scientist*, researchers measured industrial chemical levels (including DDE and PCBs) in the blood and breast milk of mothers and fetal blood from umbilical cords. Then they tracked the 600 children in the study. They found that those children who had the greatest prenatal exposure to chemicals entered puberty a full eleven months earlier than those children with the lowest exposure.[242]

LATE MENOPAUSE

Also, aside from beginning to menstruate earlier in life, women who start out on a high-fat diet and follow such a diet for their lifetime typically experience late menopause, a risk factor itself for breast cancer. Menopause usually occurs between 45 and 55, with the average age being 52. So a woman who began menstruating four years earlier and stopped menstruating four years later than the average woman has been exposed to eight additional years of heightened estrogen. This increases the risk for breast cancer and is a very serious repercussion of following the standard American diet.

START KIDS WITH A PLANT-BASED DIET

We have ample evidence to confirm that those who eat a diet based upon high-fat, low-fiber animal products have an elevated risk for a host of chronic degenerative diseases, including breast cancer. It is easier to start eating well at an early age than to have to make the sometimes difficult transition later in life, and perhaps at a time when one's health has already been severely compromised.

There is no reason not to encourage a plant-based diet.* Rest assured that a child who eats a plant-based diet will not be at any sort of developmental disadvantage, given that his or her diet is composed of a variety of whole grains, vegetables, legumes, fruits, and nuts and seeds. A recent study has confirmed once again that vegetarian children had normal growth and were even leaner than their omnivorous counterparts.[243]

START KIDS WITH ORGANIC FOODS

As indicated, pesticide residues on food pose a serious threat to adults, they pose an extraordinary risk to infants and children. One reason is that children consume proportionately far more food and water than adults. For example, an infant could consume as much as 15 times the amount of pears an adult consumes. Further, infants and children do not have near the capacity to detoxify and eliminate chemicals from their body. **According to a recent report by the Washington, D.C.-based Environmental Working Group (EWG) and**

One prime example of where children are quietly and slowly, but surely, being poisoned is at school.

---

*For further information about children and the vegan diet, please see Dr. Michael Klaper's book *Pregnancy, Children, and the Vegan Diet* (Maui: Gentle World, Inc. 1994).

based upon an analysis of federal data, every day, 1 million U.S. children age five and under consume unsafe levels of pesticides that can harm the developing brain and nervous system.[244] The report is based upon more than 80,000 samples of food tested by the U.S. Department of Agriculture (USDA) and the Food and Drug Administration, and dietary records for more than 4,000 children collected by the USDA. The foods most likely to contain unsafe levels are peaches, apples, nectarines, popcorn and pears. In the EWG study, researchers also tested baby foods produced by the 3 major US baby food suppliers. Sadly, 16 different pesticides were detected in the eight food products tested. The pesticides detected included known carcinogens, neurotoxins, endocrine disruptors as well as others with unknown effects. In baby foods, pears, peaches, and apple juice most frequently had elevated levels. The National Resources Defense Council has stated that the quantity of pesticide residues contained in commonly eaten foods during childhood may be initiating up to 6,200 cancers annually.

BABY FOOD	PESTICIDES IN BABY FOOD	
	Number of Pesticides	Health Effects
PEARS	5	Neurotoxins, endocrine disruptors
PEACHES	4	Carcinogens, neurotoxins
APPLESAUCE	4	Neurotoxins
PLUMS	3	Carcinogens, neurotoxins
SQUASH	3	Carcinogens
GREEN BEANS	3	Endocrine disruptors, neurotoxins
SWEET POTATOES	2	Effect Unknown

Source: Environmental Working Group

MINIMIZE CHILDREN'S EXPOSURE TO TOXIC CHEMICALS

The advice for avoiding toxic chemical exposure applies to children as well as to adults. The problem is that often children need adults to speak out on their behalf if such protection is to be provided. The reality is that of the 80,000 chemicals in use today, few have been tested for health effects specific to children.

One prime example of where children are quietly and slowly, but surely, being poisoned is at school. A 1997 survey of schools in California alone brought this alarming problem to light. In the survey of 46 different school districts it was found that pesticides were commonly used on playing fields, in cafeterias, classrooms, and even on school buses in an effort to combat roaches, lice, rodents, and weeds. The list of chemicals used was extensive, their possible side effects, chilling. Of the schools responding to the survey, 9 percent used chemicals that are "probable" or "known" human carcinogens, 32 percent used chemicals that are "possible" human carcinogens, 24 percent used chemicals that are developmental or reproductive toxins, 24 percent used chemicals that are known to disrupt hormone activity in the body, and 19 percent used chemicals that are classified by the EPA as Category II Nerve Toxins.[245] Even in the home, pesticide exposure is prevalent. A recent study in Florida found pesticide residues in 100 percent of the indoor air tested.[246] A study published in the November 1997 issue of Environmental Health Perspectives showed strong association between tumor development in children and the use of pesticide foggers in the home during their mother's pregnancy.

The Environmental Working Group published a study in 1993 which showed that millions of American children will be exposed to up to 35 percent of their "maximum safe lifetime dose" of pesticides by the time they are age 5. Every step should be taken to be sure this does not happen to your child.

Earlier the endocrine–disrupting substance bisphenol-A was discussed as a constituent of some plastics. It also happens to be an ingredient in a common dental sealant that is often used on children's teeth.[247] Be sure to consult with your family dentist about this before any such product is applied to your child's teeth.

AVOID POLYVINYL CHLORIDE (PVC) PRODUCTS

As stated earlier, PVC is pervasive in the environment. Composed of and vinyl chloride which has been linked to breast cancer, and ethylene dichloride, a suspected human carcinogen, PVC poses a hazard to all life, particularly to infants and children.

PVC comes to us through an amazing array of consumer products from garden hoses to credit cards, as well as products made expressly for infants and children. This includes teethers, pacifiers, plastic bathtubs and bathtub toys, and inflatable toys, as well as a variety of other things that a child may place in their mouth. Most of these items constructed using PVC also contain the toxic plastisizer known as phthalates (pronounced thalates). The most common phthalates used are di-ethylhexyl-phthalate (DEHP), di-isodecylphthalate (DIDP), and di-isononyl-phthalate.

Pthalates are not only endocrine disrupters (in humans and animals), they have been linked with cancer, kidney and liver damage, and lowered sperm counts in rats, as well as damage to the reproductive organs. Phthalates are considered a human carcinogen, as well.

Since they are not chemically bound to PVC, phthalates become mobile quite easily and can end up just about anywhere, including children's mouths. The Danish Department of Environmental Chemistry has confirmed the transfer of phthalates from teething rings sold in Denmark. Since heat assists is the leaching process, another prime opportunity for phthalate contamination is with to-go food containers. As hot, fatty food comes in contact with the container surface, phthalates can easily migrate into the food.

While other countries such as Sweden have taken the health hazards posed by PVC plastics and phthalates much more seriously, even proposing an outright ban of PVC, the U.S. has been rather sluggish in its response to the problem. Therefore, it is up to each of us to be vigilant about minimizing exposure to the compounds.

In regards to protecting children, one of the wisest things you can do is simply avoid plastic toys and products. While proponents of plastics argue that some plastic is safer than others, plastic is overwhelming our lives today, and not all of it is recyclable. In fact, PVC-based plastic is the least recyclable of all plastics in use. Plastic that can not be recycled will often end up in an incinerator which then releases dioxin into the environment. Therefore, choose toys that are made from untreated wood, metal, or natural (preferably organic) fibers. If you are truly motivated to impact the current deluge of PVC-based toys, you may wish to contact major toy manufacturers such as Mattel, Hasbro, Galoob and others, and ask what their position is on PVC and phthalates. Your expression of concern may encourage toy makers to make the switch to less harmful alternatives.

ENCOURAGE EXERCISE EARLY IN LIFE

Exercise during the reproductive years provides powerful risk reduction for breast cancer. Dr. Leslie Bernstein and colleagues at the University of Southern California found that exercise early in life in adolescence may reduce the frequency of ovulatory cycles, as well as change the length of the luteal and follicular phases of the cycle. The net result is a lowered total exposure of hormones during a particularly critical period in a woman's life.[248] Essentially, the more active women are at this stage in their life, the better off they will be, and, it appears, the lower their risk of cancer in their menopausal years. Therefore, it makes good sense that we encourage regular physical activity from an early age (before menarche), to reduce the risk of breast cancer as well as many other diseases later in life.

As parents practice the basic principles of the seven steps to breast cancer prevention with their children from birth on, the next generation will be healthier and less at risk not only for breast cancer but for other degenerative diseases. Our growing knowledge both of risk factors and of practical preventive measures offers us both a challenge and an opportunity. We owe it to our children to adopt the healthy lifestyles that will serve us all.

PART THREE

Cooking for Health
with Jean-Marc Fullsack

*"The Chinese make no distinction
between food and medicine."*

Lin Yutang

CHAPTER NINETEEN

Making the Transition

Depending on your current dietary habits, changing over to lifelong healthy eating habits initially may be a challenge. But when you consider the tremendous benefit of reducing your risk of breast cancer along with a host of other debilitating diseases and unpleasant chronic conditions, it is well worth rising to the challenge. The fact that you are reading this book in the first place is an indication that you wish to live a long, healthy life, physically fit and free of disease. Addressing only exercise gives you an incomplete equation and, therefore, provides compromised results. As you have seen, compromising in the food choices you make can ultimately have grave consequences on your health.

Substantial evidence continues to show that the wisest choice one can make regarding one's diet is to eliminate animal products

Lifelong health through nutrition and exercise comes from a lifelong commitment to making the wisest choices about what we feed our body and the way in which we exercise and care for it. Substantial evidence continues to show that the wisest choice one can make regarding one's diet is to eliminate animal products entirely.

It is understandable that for some people, changing lifelong eating patterns that have largely focused on animal products may seem an enormous challenge at first. However, as you begin to feel better, look better, have more energy, and improve your health, your new diet will become easier and easier to follow and, gradually, effortless.

Some people feel that the best way to make the transition to a vegetarian diet is to make a sweeping change all at once. They believe they should stop consuming all animal products on a particular day, and let that be that. For those who have been thinking a great deal about their diet for some time and have a very strong sense of self-discipline, this may be an effective approach. If you feel ready and have the strength, do it. You will notice dramatic changes most rapidly. However, I also recognize that such an approach can sometimes be too demanding and less successful in the long run than a gradual adaptation. In many cases, it genuinely seems more effective to make the transition gradual.

Sudden changes not only are challenging psychologically but also can be a shock to the body. As an example, people who have been consuming only a minimum of fiber in their diet may experience temporary digestive problems if they suddenly consume the recommended amount of 25 to 30 grams a day. Yet, if they gradually introduce more fiber into their diet, the transition is almost always smooth.

Again, depending on your current diet, if you were to attempt to suddenly adopt everything I have presented thus far, not only would you likely feel overwhelmed, but in fact you might even panic. So don't place that kind of pressure on yourself to begin with. Many of us have been eating the same foods in the same manner for most of our lives. We have acquired the tastes we have over time and through repetition; it is through the same repetition that we can learn new eating habits that will assure us a healthy and long life. As you make these changes, be aware of the good you are doing for yourself and how you are positively affecting your health and overall feeling of well-being. As you feel better and look better, greater change will come more easily and more naturally. You may even find yourself disliking the look, smell, and appearance of animal foods after some time, much as a smoker who quits smoking becomes sensitized to and displeased by secondhand smoke in his or her environment.

The easiest way to make the transition to the Revised American Diet™ is to do so gradually, adopting new habits one by one. By progressively weaning your body from those unhealthy foods it has come to expect and replacing those foods with healthier choices, you will permit adaptation and a chance to acquire new tastes while restoring nutritional balance. **Remember, though, since moderate changes produce moderate results, your ultimate goal is to eliminate unhealthy foods from your diet entirely.** Here is a summary of some steps you can take in making your transition:

1. Eliminate meat, poultry, and fish.

If you don't feel ready to eliminate meat entirely, start by cutting back on both the portion size and frequency with which you eat it. First, limit eating meat to no more than three times a week. When you do have meat, make it a garnish rather than the centerpiece of your meal. For example, rather than having a steak or a couple of chicken breasts, mince a bit of turkey and mix it with a larger portion of rice and vegetables. Begin incorporating tofu, tofu and veggie burgers, and tofu hot dogs, as well as tempeh products, into your meals.

2. Eliminate dairy products.

If you are not ready to eliminate dairy products entirely, begin by switching to nonfat or skim milk products. This will cut back considerably on fat content. Remember, whole milk contains nearly 50 percent of its calories as fat. Low-fat milk has about 38 percent of its calories as fat. Many people erroneously believe that 2 percent milk is 2 percent fat. Unfortunately, this is not the case. Indeed, 2 percent milk still gets 22 percent of its calories from fat. However, skim or nonfat milk gets only 4 percent of its calories from fat.

During this transition period, choose organic dairy products. Begin using soy milk, rice milk, oat milk, or almond milk. These great-tasting replacements can be used just like milk on cold or hot cereals and in your favorite recipes that call for milk. Soy milks and other non-dairy beverages are sold in 8-ounce aseptic containers that needn't be refrigerated until they are opened. They are available in tasty flavors such as chocolate, mocha, and vanilla. You can substitute mashed tofu in recipes that call for ricotta or cottage cheese. Although soy cheeses are often recommended to the cheese lover, be aware that this alternative product may contain casein, a cow's milk protein. The protein is added to soy cheese to give it the "stretchy" consistency as it melts. Even ice cream and other yummy frozen desserts made from soybeans, rice, and fruit are available.

3. Eliminate your intake of eggs.

By eliminating eggs, you will eliminate one of the most concentrated sources of cholesterol in the diet. At first, you may wish to limit your use of eggs to no more that three a week. Try removing at least one egg yolk, as this is the primary source of cholesterol and saturated fat. In place of scrambled eggs in the morning, you may opt to try some of the egg-replacement products available. Better yet, in place of eggs for breakfast, try the delicious scrambled tofu recipe in Chapter 21.

4. Eliminate refined flours, grains, and sugars.

By eliminating refined sugars from your diet, you will enjoy a restored balance in energy and lose the terrible cravings that are associated with a diet high in refined sugars. In place of refined sugar, you may wish to try barley malt syrup, brown rice syrup, and turbinado date sugar. These sweeteners can be found at most natural foods markets. In place of sweets, rely on fresh fruit. You can be sure that anytime you order a plate of pasta in a restaurant, it will be made from refined white flour. The exception, of course, is when the menu indicates that the pasta is made from whole-wheat flour. So when you purchase pasta in the market, look for "whole wheat" on the package. It is much the same with rice. If a restaurant gives you the option, choose the brown rice over the white. By choosing brown rice over polished white rice you will enjoy a richer source of vitamins, minerals, and natural bran, as well as a more hearty flavor. The same benefits come from choosing whole-wheat flour over refined white flour. Choose whole-wheat breads, rolls, muffins, and tortillas, too.

5. Eliminate butter, margarine, mayonnaise, and oils.

Butter, margarine, and mayonnaise, what I call "luxury fats," are rich in saturated fat, dangerous trans-fats, and cholesterol. It is important that you cut back on your consumption of these foods. Soon you will really begin to taste the breads you may have previously smothered in butter. In place of butter and margarine, try apple butter, unsweetened fruit spreads, and nut butters.

Limit your use of vegetable oil. If you choose to use any oil at all, my recommendation is that it be extra virgin olive oil made from cold-pressed, organic olives and then bottled in green glass. In place of oil, you can steam vegetables or use vegetable stock or soy-based "chicken" broth to cook and sauté vegetables or to prepare other dishes.

6. Increase your intake of fresh, organic vegetables and fruits, legumes and whole grains.

For their abundance of fiber and density of antioxidant vitamins, minerals, and cancer-fighting phytochemicals, choose fresh vegetables and fruits more often. For variety, include new fruits and vegetables you haven't tried. Have fruit salad for breakfast, make fruit smoothies, and carry fruit with you as an "anytime snack." Try to consume most of your fruit whole rather than juiced. Whole fruit retains its important fiber, and its natural sugars are assimilated more slowly. As juice, fruit sugars can be assimilated too quickly. (You can dilute the concentration of juices by "halving" them with water).

Use vegetables in pasta, steamed over rice, in a marinara, or as a main dish vegetable "stir–fry." Cut up vegetables and fruit in advance to keep them handy as a snack throughout the day, and store washed and cut fruits and vegetables in the fridge to make your next meal preparation quick and easy.

Try hot oatmeal or quinoa with fresh fruit, cinnamon and nutmeg for a yummy breakfast dish. Experiment with cous cous, amaranth, buckwheat and the many other grains to choose from.

Incorporate black beans, navy beans, lentils, and other legumes into your meals often.

You will probably find that after about a month of following the Revised American Diet,™ you will have successfully overcome the urge to slip backwards and consume unhealthy animal products as well as foods high in sodium and refined sugars. After only two weeks, you will have naturally lost unwanted body weight, show markedly better-looking skin, and feel more energized throughout the day. You may notice that symptoms like chronic congestion, persistent headaches, gas, and indigestion seem to vanish. You will probably find that you need less sleep and wake up feeling rejuvenated rather than sluggish. If you have been taking medications, you may find that they are no longer necessary (although always check with your physician before

After only two weeks, you will have naturally lost unwanted body weight, show markedly better-looking skin, and feel more energized throughout the day.

making any changes). If you have your cholesterol and blood pressure checked prior to making the transition and then again in two months, you will likely see a continuing decrease in both.

Basic Steps in Overcoming the Standard American Diet

1. Eliminate meat, poultry, and fish.
2. Eliminate dairy products.
3. Eliminate your intake of eggs.
4. Eliminate refined flours, grains, and sugars.
5. Eliminate butter, margarine, mayonnaise, and oils.
6. Increase your intake of fresh, organic vegetables and fruits, legumes, and whole grains.

FOOD ADDITIVES TO AVOID

Reading the labels on food packaging is another step you can take to safeguard your health. For example, take a look at the ingredient label of your favorite sandwich bread. You might be surprised to find hydrogenated oil listed as an ingredient. As previously mentioned, hydrogenated oil is your warning that the product contains trans fatty acids which are linked with cancer. There are plenty of delicious and nutritious whole-grain breads available without this dangerous additive. Other ingredient you should watch out for include the following:

Artificial color

It is not uncommon for artificial colors to cause allergic reactions in people. It is believed that the coloring Yellow No. 5 can worsen the condition of asthmatics. According to the Center for Science in the Public Interest (CSPI), Blue No. 1 and No. 2, and Green No. 3 have all been linked to cancer in animals. **According to a study in *Environmental Health Perspectives*, Red No. 3 can bind to hormone receptors in the breasts and cause DNA damage and thereby instigate cancer.**[249]

Aspartame

A sweetener manufactured from methanol (wood alcohol) and two amino acids, Aspartame is sold under the names Equal® and Nutrasweet®, and has been linked to literally thousands of health problems. In fact, the FDA has logged over 3,000 complaints about this product, with symptoms including headache, numbness, dizziness, nausea, depression, and vision problems. Those who suffer from phenylketonuria (PKU), individuals who cannot break down the amino acid phenylalanine, must avoid this product and those products in which it is contained.

Butylated Hydroxyanisole (BHA)

BHA is a preservative that is commonly found in packaged foods, including baked goods, soups, potato flakes, breakfast cereals, and chewing gum. This product may have adverse effects on the nervous system.

Butylated Hydroxytoluene (BHT)

BHT is used similarly to BHA. It is believed to be toxic to the kidneys, and has the additional risk of being a suspected carcinogen. The United Kingdom has already banned the use of this additive.

Mono- and Diglycerides

These are chemical preservatives commonly used in breads, frozen desserts, margarine, conventional peanut butter, and numerous baked goods. They are currently being studied for adverse reproductive effects.

Propyl Gallate

A preservative used similarly to BHA and BHT, this additive may cause stomach and skin irritation and is a suspected carcinogen. It is used in ice cream, some fruit drinks, candy, and gelatin desserts. Those who have asthma are particularly sensitive to it.

Saccharin

Saccharin is an artificial sweetener that the FDA has considered banning for some years now. A known carcinogen, it still shows up in some soft drinks and in Sweet 'N Low® brand sweetener.

Sodium Nitrite

Commonly used in bacon, ham, smoked fish and sandwich meats, this preservative is a known carcinogen.

DINING OUT

Eating at restaurants as a vegetarian is much easier that you might think. These days there is a heightened awareness of different eating concerns, and not only are restaurants willing to be accommodating but some also cater specifically to vegetarians.

In almost any restaurant, you should have no problem asking for a plate of steamed vegetables and brown rice.* You can also always order a meal-sized salad and request that dressings be served on the side. In place of dressing, ask for a few lemon wedges to squeeze over your greens. Better yet, bring your own favorite dressing with you. Many restaurants also offer full salad bars where you can find an abundance of vegetables such as broccoli, cucumbers, onions, celery, peppers, tomatoes, carrots, and sprouts. Be careful when choosing a dressing from these bars, however.

Most often they serve commercial dressings that not only contain eggs and milk products but also are extremely high in both sodium and sugar.

Most often they serve commercial dressings that not only contain eggs and milk products but also are extremely high in both sodium and sugar.

Italian restaurants have an abundance of pasta dishes from which to choose. If you see one you'd like that is prepared with cream sauce, simply ask your waiter to substitute a marinara or classic red sauce. Polenta, a coarse cornmeal, is also often found on the menus of Italian restaurants, usually served with a marinara or vegetable sauce. Another common dish is risotto (rice), often made with saffron and mixed vegetables.

Chinese restaurants can be another haven for vegetarian diners. Many of their dishes are centered on vegetables and rice. You will also find tofu dishes. Unfortunately, some Chinese restaurants continue to use MSG as a seasoning. Not only is this a source of sodium, but some people have allergic reactions to it. Also, salt and oil are often used liberally in the preparation of Chinese dishes. Ask your waiter if your dish can be prepared without these three items. Steamed vegetables are usually an option.

At Mexican restaurants, you can always ask for a hearty vegetarian burrito made from rice, beans, salsa, and vegetables. Be sure to request that they hold the cheese, since it is often automatically added to burritos. Ask your wait person if the restaurant uses lard or oils in the preparation of its beans. Neither of these will be a healthy addition to what is otherwise a nutritious meal.

*For a directory of natural foods restaurants, stores, and distributors, please visit
http://www.naturalfoodsdirectory.com

At Middle Eastern restaurants you can choose from a variety of vegetable, grain, and legume dishes. A popular dish is Yalanji Yaprak, which is baked eggplant stuffed with vegetables. Another healthful dish is couscous, which is steamed bulgur wheat, served with vegetables.

Even in the worst situations you usually have a choice. Many of today's fast-food establishments are providing hearty baked potatoes stuffed with broccoli or cauliflower and offer salad bars to complement the meal.

If you have been invited to eat at a friend's house, let your hosts know that you are a vegetarian so they have time to prepare for you. Some people have told me that it makes them uncomfortable, thinking that explaining that they are vegetarian is demanding or rude. On the contrary, I have found that people would much rather know what my preferences are in advance and try to accommodate them rather than see me avoiding their food later. You can always offer to bring your favorite dish. If you are not yet comfortable with your new vegetarian lifestyle and/or believe that your host might be hurt by your desire not to eat certain foods, you can always say that you have an allergy or are under the strict orders of your doctor.

The bottom line, however, is that it is *your* health at stake and that is what is most important. Author Victoria Moran put it succinctly when she said, "You can say no to any food offered you by any person on this planet. If that person is offended, there's a problem, but the problem isn't yours."

CHAPTER TWENTY

Staple Foods of the Revised American Diet™

In this chapter, we continue to examine the basic components of a healthy diet, which for current purposes I have dubbed the Revised American Diet.™ By keeping your kitchen stocked with these healthy foods, as well as using care when you eat out, you'll be well on your way to adopting a healthy lifestyle that maximizes your chances of preventing breast cancer.

FRUITS, VEGETABLES, GRAINS, AND LEGUMES

Aside from the wonderfully sweet tastes they offer, fruits, along with vegetables, are one of the primary sources of cancer-preventive antioxidants, fiber, and phytochemicals.

Those who consume five servings of fruits and vegetables a day cut their cancer risk by about 50 percent. **In fact, to date, over 125 studies have confirmed the cancer preventive power of a diet rich in fruits and vegetables.**[250] For many Americans, vegetables are used to "garnish" a plate of beef, chicken, or other main dish. Many of us also fixate on certain vegetables. For instance, tomatoes and carrots are popular, but what about the abundance of other vegetables available to us? Since vegetables offer us important vitamins, minerals, phytochemicals, and fiber, all essential components of health, they should make up a large part of the meals we eat. Consider just how many other colorful, tasty vegetables there are to choose from: artichokes, asparagus, beets, broccoli, Brussels sprouts, cabbage, cauliflower, chard, cucumber, eggplant, green beans, greens, jicama, kale, leeks, lettuce, mushrooms, onions, peppers, potatoes, pumpkin, spinach, squash, and sweet potatoes.

Fruit is rich in vitamins (particularly A and C) and minerals (magnesium, copper, and manganese) and high in fiber. One medium orange contains over 60 mg of vitamin C. A small persimmon offers 218 mg of vitamin C. One cup of raisins contains 102 mg of calcium and 2 mg of iron. An average serving of cantaloupe offers over half the recommended daily intake of vitamin A. Bananas provide a substantial supply of potassium.

The sweetness of fruit comes from a natural form of sugar, unlike the sugars found in many processed sweets such as cookies, candies, and soft drinks. The sugar in fruit provides the body with a more balanced supply of energy. Those fruits highest in fiber are apples, apricots, oranges, bananas, peaches, pears, and raisins. Fruits also contain a high quantity of water, something most of us could use more of.

Some individuals experience digestive difficulties when they combine fruit with other foods. If you have this experience, make a point of eating your fruits separately, such as early in the morning at least a half-hour before breakfast and as between-meal snacks.

FOOD GROUP	EXAMPLES FROM THE FOUR FOOD GROUPS
WHOLE GRAINS	Amaranth, barley, buckwheat, bulgur, quinoa, millet, rye, triticale, rye, pasta, cereals (oatmeal, granola and shredded wheat), breads, tortillas, corn, popcorn, cornmeal, cornflour, brown rice, oats, spelt, kamut.
VEGETABLES	Artichokes, asparagus, bamboo shoots, beets, broccoli, brussel sprouts, babbage, barrots, cauliflower, chard, cucumber, garlic, eggplant, jicama, kale, leeks, parsley, sprouts, lettuce, peas, peppers, pumpkin, onions, tomatoes, mushrooms, potatoes, spinach, squash,yams.
LEGUMES	Adzuki beans, black beans, cranberry beans, fava beans, flageolets, great Northern beans, kidney beans, lima beans, mung beans, navy beans, pinto beans, red beans, soybeans, black-eyed peas, chickpeas, red lentils, green split peas, yellow split peas, brown lentils, green lentils, tempeh, tofu, soy milk.
FRUITS	Apples, blackberries, cranberries, guavas, mangoes, peaches, pineapples, apricots, blueberries, figs, kiwis, melons, pears, raisins, bananas, boysenberries, grapefruits, lemons, oranges, plums, raspberries, dates, cherries, limes, papayas, prunes, strawberries.

Grains

Around the world, grains have played an important part in the diet of many societies. For instance, in Central America, corn has been a dietary mainstay, while in the Middle East, millet is eaten regularly. In North Africa, couscous is popular, and in Italy, people enjoy polenta. In Asia, rice and bulgur wheat are staples, and in Scotland, oats.

Whole grains are a rich source of fiber, vitamins (particularly B and E), and minerals (particularly magnesium, calcium, and iron) and are an excellent source of complex carbohydrates. Unfortunately, the average American eats very few whole-grain foods. Oddly enough, while we are the largest producer of grain in the world, over half our grain production is used for livestock feed.

A major drawback of the grain consumed in America is that it has often been processed in a way that compromises its nutritional quality. Before they are refined, grains are composed of germ, bran, and endosperm. Some grains may also contain an outer shell called the hull. During the milling process, however, most of the bran, vitamins, and minerals are lost.

As an example, let's look at flour. All flour begins in a whole form. However, after a process of grinding, rolling, and sifting the grain, the seed is separated. What is retained is the "powdered" endosperm. This endosperm is then bleached (with chemicals such as benzoyl peroxide, or acetone peroxide) and finally becomes the common white flour you find in the supermarket. When whole-wheat flour is made, all components of the

NUTRIENT	NUTRIENT COMPARISON	
	Whole Wheat Flour	Enriched White Flour
FIBER	11.6 g	3.5 g
CALCIUM	50 mg	20 mg
PHOSPHOROUS	445 mg	100 mg
MAGNESIUM	135 mg	30 mg
ZINC	2.9 mg	0.8 mg
VITAMIN B_6	1.1 mg	0.07 mg
PANTOTHENIC ACID	1.3 mg	0.5 mg
FOLIC ACID	46 mcg	20 mcg

Nutrient comparison of one cup whole wheat flour and one cup enriched white flour.

seed are retained and recombined after milling. In refined white flours, over 50 percent of the vitamins and nearly 25 percent of the fiber can be lost, leaving you with a fraction of the original nutritional value.

This is why when shopping for breads you should make sure the label says, "whole wheat." Without the word whole, the bread could be made from a mix of refined and whole grains, or colored, processed grains. The word whole is your assurance that the product still contains the bran and germ of the grain.

Grains are refined for three reasons. First, the process makes some grains easier to eat. Second, it makes the grain cook faster. Finally, when a grain is refined, the natural oil content is removed. Food manufacturers prefer not to have the oil present because it reduces the shelf life of the grain. To make up for the lost nutrients, food manufacturers will "enrich" processed foods with certain vitamins and minerals; yet, as Table 2 illustrates, enriched grains will never equal the nutritional quality of whole grains.

Another problem with the enriching process is that the nutrients may be inadvertently washed away. Most enriched grains are "sprayed" with nutrient-containing formula. However, rinsing the grain or using excessive water when cooking can wash away these nutrients. This problem occurs most often with rice, because it is often thoroughly rinsed prior to cooking, a procedure that can result in a reduction of up to 50 percent of the nutrients that were sprayed on.

The best way to eat grains is in their whole and natural form. This way you will be assured of receiving all the naturally occurring nutrients as well as the health-promoting bran. Let's look at the numerous grains you have to choose from.

Amaranth

Amaranth's history dates back to the Aztecs. Today, amaranth is produced largely in China and Central America. This tiny, pale yellow grain can be used like wheat. In cooking, you can split a wheat-flour measurement, using half amaranth and half wheat flour. Amaranth has a high protein content and is richer in calcium than any other grain.

Barley

Barley was first cultivated in China around 2000 B.C. Today, the most popular form of barley is an ivory-colored form called "pearled barley," which has its bran removed. The most nutritious form is "hulled barley," in which the bran is left intact and the fiber, iron, and calcium content remains high. Barley is also a rich source of potassium. This versatile grain can be added to soups, broth, and salads, mixed with vegetables, and even made into a hot breakfast cereal.

Buckwheat

Technically, buckwheat is not a grain because it is not part of the gramineae grass family. Nevertheless, this food is loaded with vitamin E, potassium, phosphorus, and B vitamins. With the exception of "buckwheat pancakes," this grain has not enjoyed much popularity in the United States, which is quite a loss. Buckwheat has a distinct taste and a rich, nutty flavor.

Cornmeal

A staple for the Native Americans, cornmeal is made from ground corn. Like other grains, the best way to buy it is in its whole form with the germ and bran still present. While most people have had cornbread and corn muffins, this hearty grain can make terrific pancakes and can be made into polenta, a dish that is increasing in popularity in the United States.

Kamut

Once known as "King Tut's wheat," this buttery-flavored grain is a relative of modern wheat. Kamut is higher in protein than many other grains and rich in minerals. An increasing number of organic Kamut breads, cereals, and pastas are available.

Millet

Considered a sacred food by the Chinese, millet is high in protein, the B vitamins, copper, and iron. The grain is small and absorbs flavors well. Like barley, millet can be made into a tasty hot cereal. It can also be mixed into salads or casseroles or eaten in place of rice. Those who make their own granola at home may enjoy adding millet to the mix.

Oats

Oats contain calcium, phosphorus, iron, vitamin E, thiamin, riboflavin, and the B-vitamin complex. Although oats have been around for almost 2,000 years and have always been a primary staple in the diet of the Scottish, they didn't gain popularity in the United States until recently. This interest has been brought about by numerous publicized studies that show that oat bran can play an important part in lowering cholesterol levels.

Fortunately, all oats retain their bran and germ, so their fiber content is higher than grains that have been refined. Of all the grains, oats seem to be the most popular for making hot cereal (oatmeal), either old-fashioned or quick-cooking. The old-fashioned variety comprises whole oats that have been heated and rolled flat. Quick-cooking oats have been sliced and then heated and rolled; this process makes them cook in about a minute. Granola, which has become quite popular, is also made from oats.

Oats can be used to make healthy and hearty muffins. If you make your own breads, try adding oats to the recipe. For a heartier and flavorful pancake, add oats to your whole-wheat cakes!

Quinoa

Pronounced *keen-wah*, this staple of the Incas is quickly becoming very popular in the United States. Known as a "super nutrient" grain, quinoa is packed with iron, riboflavin, manganese, zinc, copper, potassium, and magnesium. It has a pale yellow color when cooked and a mild, nutty flavor. Quinoa works well mixed in most baked goods and can be a great addition to a green salad.

Rice

There are numerous varieties of rice, including long-grain, short-grain, white, brown, wehani, wild, arborio, and basmati. Although rice is the most popular grain food in the United States, this country is at the bottom of the list in terms of world consumption. In Asia, the nutritional value of rice has long been known, and the grain is a primary staple of the Asian diet.

Rice is a good source of B vitamins, iron, magnesium, and phosphorus, as well as protein. Like barley, however, the bulk of rice eaten in the United States is in the refined form of polished white rice. Conversely, brown rice retains its bran and germ and is considerably richer in vitamins, minerals, and fiber.

Rye

One of the least known grains, rye is significantly higher in protein than whole wheat. It also contains B vitamins and iron. While consumed widely in Scandinavia, what little rye we eat in the United States is in the form of rye bread, which is largely refined wheat flour and rye mixed together. Rye can be added to oatmeal, bread, muffins, and rice or, in its flake form, prepared as a hot cereal or mixed in with homemade granola.

Spelt

This 5,000-year-old grain is becoming quite popular, particularly among those who have gluten and other grain allergies,* because of its low gluten level. It has a nutty flavor and is rich in B vitamins. Recently, several spelt breads and bagels have been introduced by alternative baking companies.

LEGUMES

A legume is a plant that bears seeds enclosed in pods that split upon maturity. We eat these pods in the form of beans, peas, and lentils. Legumes are probably the oldest crop in the world. Some evidence has indicated that they may have been an important crop as far back as 10,000 years ago. Today legumes make up a substantial part of the diet of people in Asia, Latin America, the Middle East, and India.

Until recently legumes were an ignored food source in America. They have been called the "poor man's protein." The truth is that they are an outstanding, inexpensive, and very versatile food that provides not only a significant amount of protein (12-20 grams per cup) and fiber (6-8 grams per cup) but also a substantial supply of the B vitamins, calcium, magnesium, iron, potassium, and zinc, as well as several anti cancer phytochemicals. Another wonderful quality of legumes is that they are extremely durable and store well. Stored in a well-sealed container in a dry place, legumes can be kept for up to a year.

In Asia, soy makes up a large part of the diet—fifty times as much as in the typical American diet—and rates for breast and prostate cancer are very low.

Most varieties of legumes are delicious eaten alone or as a side dish, added to soups or chilies, combined with rice, or mixed with a variety of vegetables. One of the reasons that legumes have not been as popular as they could be is the myth that they are difficult to cook. On the contrary, legumes are one of the easiest foods to prepare.

Soy Foods

Soy beans, and the foods made from them can aptly be called miracle foods. Not only has it been shown that tofu and other soy foods contain phytochemicals — including isoflavones (genistein and diadzein), protease

---

*An excellent cookbook for those who are contending with food allergies is *The Feel Good Food Guide* by Deborah Page Johnson, (Naperville: New Page Productions, 1996).

inhibitors, and phytic acids — that not only provide protection from heart disease, osteoporosis, and certain forms of cancer, but also, numerous studies have demonstrated the cholesterol-lowering effect of soy. Even hot flashes have been mitigated through soy in the diet.

Soy Reduces Risk of Breast and Other Cancers

In Asia, soy makes up a large part of the diet — fifty times as much as in the typical American diet — and rates for breast and prostate cancer are very low. Yet, you don't have to live in Asia to benefit from soy. Studies have shown that women in the U.S. who consume soy regularly have about a 50 percent reduced risk of breast cancer when compared to the general population.[251] Some studies have suggested that as little as a cup of soy milk or a half-cup of tofu a day can sharply reduce risk.[252] A study of Singapore women with and without breast cancer found that the cancer-free women ate about 55 grams of soy a day.[253]

As mentioned earlier, genestein, just one important isoflavone in soy, seems to interfere with angiogenesis,[254] the process whereby new blood vessels are established. Without these vessels bringing in oxygen and nutrients, the tumors are effectively starved to death before they have a chance to metastasize to other organs of the body.[255] Genestein also increases the production of sex-hormone-binding globulin (SHBG).[256] This carrier molecule is responsible for keeping estrogens bound and "out of play." When SHBG levels are lower, as they are in individuals who follow a high-fat diet, more estrogens are left free where they can elevate risk.

Some research indicates that genestein may also play a role in suppressing skin cancer (melanoma) cells.[257] Currently, research is focusing on whether soy foods can block metastasis from occurring entirely in an established cancer.[258]

Phytoestrogens

When converted by enzymes from intestinal bacteria, these isoflavones yield a weak estrogen quality. Researchers believe that the weak plant estrogen is able to occupy hormone receptors on breast cells and other tissue. By doing so, the plant estrogen displaces the body's more potent estrogen that would otherwise be able to occupy the receptor and potentially heighten risk of cancer.

Different Needs, Different Effect

It seems that the effect of plant estrogens is different according to a woman's need. In premenopausal women, whose hormone production is higher, plant estrogens can suppress estrogen levels enough to alter activity in both the breast and uterine tissues, and thereby provide protection. In postmenopausal women, whose hormone production is lower, these weak plant estrogens seem to be effective at reducing the degree to which women experience postmenopausal symptoms such as hot flashes, mood swings, and vaginal dryness, all the while still protecting breast and uterine tissues.

Soy, Cholesterol Levels, and Heart Disease

Studies have also demonstrated the powerful cholesterol-lowering effect of soy when consuming as little as 25 grams a day. One recent study in the *New England Journal of Medicine* demonstrated in some cases a reduction in cholesterol of up to 20 percent in a month! Such a drop in cholesterol levels equals almost a 30 percent reduction in risk of coronary heart disease. What's more, it seems that soy foods have the effect of lowering LDL ("bad") cholesterol while not adversely affecting HDL ("good") cholesterol.

Finally, soy foods such as tofu can be a rich source of the calcium that is essential to bone integrity, and therefore, it can play an important role in reducing risk of osteoporosis when other risk factors are accounted for (See Chapter 8 for detailed information on osteoporosis risk factors).

Soy and Hot Flashes

A fascinating study conducted in Australia has shown that adding 40 grams of soy a day to the diet can reduce hot flashes. In the study, 47 women experiencing hot flashes benefited from a 40 percent reduction in this menopausal side effect. The reduction occurred in as little as six weeks![259]

While all soy foods mentioned below contain isoflavones, their content of these beneficial compounds varies according to the way in which they were grown and processed. See the following chart for reported averages of isoflavone content of selected soy foods.

SOY FOOD	AVERAGE ISOFLAVONE CONTENT
	per 3.5 oz.
ROASTED SOYBEANS	162 mg
TVP	138 mg
SOY FLOUR	112 mg
TEMPEH	62 mg
TOFU	34 mg
TOFU YOGURT	16 mg
SOY HOT DOG	15 mg
SOY NOODLES	9 mg

Tofu

Although tofu has been around for over 1,000 years in parts of Asia, in the West we are just beginning to understand the nutritional value of this versatile food. Ironically, the United States is the largest producer of soybeans (which are used to make tofu), yet we export the majority of it to other countries.

Tofu falls under the legume category and is made by curding soybean milk. Not only is it a good source of complete protein (it contains all of the essential amino acids), but it also it contains no cholesterol and, when made with calcium sulfate, is an excellent source of calcium. Furthermore, it's very affordable! While regular tofu does contain a fair amount of fat, the fat in tofu is unsaturated and, because tofu is a plant it contains no cholesterol. There are a few brands of "lite" tofu, such as Mori-Nu Lite®, that contain only a few grams of fat.

Tofu works well in almost any dish, particularly those in which you might normally include meat or poultry, such as curries or pastas; it also does wonders for homemade salad dressings. An added benefit is that many brands of tofu are made from organic soybeans.

Tempeh

Tempeh (pronounced tem-pay) is another food derived from fermented soybeans and, occasionally, grains. It is very popular in Indonesia. It has a nutty flavor and unique texture that makes it a good replacement for meat in chili and for grilling or steaming, as well as a tasty addition to vegetable sautés and pasta dishes. There are also a number of tempeh burgers on the market. Tempeh can be found either refrigerated, usually along with tofu, or frozen.

Texturized Vegetable Protein (TVP)

TVP is made from defatted soy flour that has been compressed until it takes on a flake texture. Once rehydrated, TVP works wonders in replacing the meat normally found in dishes such as chili, sloppy joes, hamburgers, and hot dogs.

Soy Flour

Soy flour is made from roasted soybeans that have been ground into a fine powder. Available in full-fat and defatted versions, soy flour is heavier than wheat flour. For this reason, it is best to limit it to 15 percent to 20 percent of a recipe's flour requirement. It can also be added to gravies and sauces.

Soy Milk

Soy milk is made by pressing soaked and cooked soybeans with water. The result is a creamy milk-like beverage with a nutty flavor that can be used in a variety of ways. Soy milk works well over cold and hot cereals, in soups and sauces, and in pancakes and other recipes that call for milk. Aside from its supply of protein and B vitamins, most soy milks are fortified with vitamins A and D, calcium, and at least one company offers vitamin B_{12} fortification.

The staple foods outlined in this chapter represent a beginning. With each small step you take toward eating more of them, you help to decrease your risk for breast cancer.

General Guidelines for The Revised American Diet™

At the end of this section you will find a chart containing serving and proportion suggestions. This is a guide and not meant to restrict you to an exact measurement of food each day. One of the pleasures of choosing a plant-based diet is that you needn't have a calculator on hand when you eat. In other words, you need not concern yourself with ratios, percentages, or grams of anything. Nor do you need to be concerned with protein combining or other food "balancing acts." Such irritations are a thing of the past. When you choose foods from the Revised American Diet™, you can, within reason, eat as much as you wish, when you wish.

In Chapter 21 you will find guidelines for stocking your kitchen with foods and ingredients essential to healthful cooking and eating. You will also find handy charts showing the best way to prepare healthful grains and legumes. Finally, in Chapter 22 you will find a fourteen-day menu plan with recipes to help get you started on the road to healthful cooking. You will even find wonderful and easy menus for holiday occasions.

As you become familiar with the foods and cooking methods described, you will probably begin formulating some of your own favorite dishes. Welcome to a whole new world of healthful foods!

FOOD GROUP	THE REVISED AMERICAN DIET ™	
	Servings per day	Serving size
WHOLE GRAINS	5 or more	1/2 cup oats (cooked) 1/2 cup brown rice (cooked) 1 cup whole-wheat pasta 1 cup cereal 1 slice bread
VEGETABLES	3 or more	1/2 cup broccoli (cooked) 1/2 cup carrots (cooked) 1/2 cup spinach/collards/kale 1 medium baked potato
LEGUMES	2-3	1/2 cup lentils (cooked) 1/2 cup black beans (cooked) 1/2 cup tofu 1 cup soy milk
FRUITS	3 or more	1 medium apple 1/2 cup chopped fruit 1/2 cup berries 1/4 cup dried fruit

Number of servings and serving sizes are provided as an initial guide. You need not be overly concerned with exact portions of whole grains, vegetables, legumes, and fruits. Some highly active individuals, such as athletes, may need more servings to maintain their body weight.

CHAPTER TWENTY-ONE

Stocking the Kitchen

As you make the transition to the Revised American Diet™, there are a number of things you will want to have on hand for preparing meals. Following are suggestions for both transitional foods as well as staples you will want to have on hand for preparing healthful meals.

Grains
Whole wheat flour
Brown rice
Oats
Quinoa
Spelt
Kamut brand wheat
Amaranth
Buckwheat

Sweeteners
Stevia*
Rice syrup
Honey
FruitSource®

Beverages
Soy milk
Rice milk
Oat milk
Almond milk
Herbal teas

Nuts & Seeds
Cashews
Almonds
Pistachios

---

*Stevia is a centuries-old natural sweetener that is widely used in Japan. It is reported that Stevia crystals are calorie-free, do not raise blood sugar levels or promote tooth decay. Stevia can be found in most natural foods markets.

Fruits
Apples
Blackberries
Cranberries
Guava
Peaches
Pineapple
Blueberries
Figs
Kiwis
Melons
Pears
Bananas
Grapefruit
Oranges
Raspberries
Cherries
Strawberries
Apple sauce

Legumes
Adzuki beans
Black beans
Fava beans
Kidney beans
Navy beans
Pinto beans
Soybeans
Chickpeas
Lentils
Split peas
Tempeh
Tofu
T.V.P

Vegetables
Broccoli
Asparagus
Brussel sprouts
Cabbage
Carrots
Cauliflower
Cucumbers
Chard
Eggplant
Garlic
Kale
Peppers
Pumpkin
Onions
Tomatoes
Potatoes
Spinach
Squash
Yams

Breakfast Cereals
Arrowhead Mills (organic)
Health Valley (organic)
Kashi Company
Nature's Path
Pacific Grain Products

Pasta Sauces
Enrico's
Garden Valley
Millina's Finest
Muir Glen
Whole Foods

Flours
Arrowhead Mills (assorted)

Non-Dairy Mayonnaise Spreads (made from tofu)
Vegenaise
Nayonaise

Ingredients for Cooking and Baking

Rumford non-aluminum
  baking powder
Shari's organic canned pumpkin
Eden organic canned black, pinto
  and chili beans
Spice Island spices
Salt and salt substitutes
Spectrum Naturals cold-pressed
  organic olive oil
Soy sauce
Tamari sauce
Rice vinegar
Muir Glenn canned, organic
  tomatoes, tomato sauce
Muir Glenn bar-b-q sauce
Falafel mix
Hain Vegetable Broth
Health Valley Vegetable Broth
Tomato salsa
Soymage "cheese topping"
Soyco, "cheese topping"

Snack Foods

Mochi, various flavors
Fresh, organic fruit
Cascadian Farms organic frozen
  fruit (for smoothies)
Govinda's Bliss bars
Lundberg organic rice cakes
Organic air popped corn
White Wave soy yogurt

Meat Substitutes

Yves Veggie Deli Slices
Yves Veggie Tofu Wieners
Yves Veggie Burger
Boca Burger
White Wave Tempeh Burger

Potato and Corn Chips (Baked)

Barbara's
Bearitos
Guiltless Gourmet
Garden of Eatin'

Fruit Spreads

Knudsen Organic Jams
Apple butter
Cascadian Farms fruit spread

IDEAS FOR DESSERT

Fresh fruit

Branch out and try some of the incredible variety of fruit available to us. Apples and oranges are great, but be sure to include peaches, pears, blueberries and kiwi fruit. Or, mix a few different kinds of fruit together for a tasty fruit salad.

Rice Dream "ice cream"

Rice Dream is a popular ice cream replacement. It is a non-dairy, frozen dessert that has a remarkable taste and texture. Rice Dream is available in many of your favorite ice cream flavors.

Rice Dream pudding

The makers of Rice Dream, Imagine Foods, have also come up with a non-dairy (rice based) pudding in tasty flavors. These make a handy snack or dessert for those who miss pudding.

Non-dairy fruit sorbet

There are many fruit sorbets available today in supermarkets. Some brands are organic. My favorite is Cascadian Farms brand. All of their fruit sorbets are dairy-free and made from organic fruit.

Lundberg's rice pudding

Lundberg is a popular name when it comes to rice, especially in California. The Lundberg family has come up with their own version of rice pudding. This is an excellent tasting dessert that can be made quickly with either soy or rice milk.

Tapioca made with soy or rice milk

Once a favorite dessert, tapioca has been forgotten by many Americans. Made from the cassava root, tapioca can be purchased in the baking good section of most markets. Usually there is a simple recipe on the box. Made with soy milk or rice dream and a little vanilla, this makes a thick and creamy dessert you'll love.

Remember, as you begin to stock up on the items mentioned in this chapter, you are taking the most important step you can take to reduce the risk of breast cancer and other deadly diseases. In the process, you may find yourself enjoying the wonderful new tastes, shapes, smells, and textures that this dietary plan can bring to you.

TIPS ON TOFU

As you will see, many of the recipes provided in the following section use tofu. As has been shown, the health benefits of soy foods are just too great to be ignored. What follows are some suggestions and guidelines for buying tofu to make these and other recipes.

Remember that aside from the recipes that are provided, you are encouraged to incorporate soy into your own recipes. Tofu is one of the most versatile foods for doing so. The great thing about tofu is that it will absorb just
about any flavor with which it is prepared.

In Japan it is estimated that there are over 30,000 different stores selling
nothing but tofu. Things are a little different in the U.S. Depending on
where you live, there may be a local tofu producer who brings tofu to your
neighborhood market. Such tofu is often found in the dairy section, either
in individually wrapped containers, or bulk, in self-serve basins of water.
This type of tofu is quite perishable and must be kept submerged in water.
If you change the water daily, it can keep about five days when refrigerated
at home.

Another convenient way to buy tofu is in aseptic containers found on
most U.S. supermarket shelves. Tofu packaged in this manner can be
purchased in advance and stored in your cupboard, ready for use, for up to
a year. Be sure to check the date stamp on the package.

Soft Tofu

Soft tofu has a custard–like texture that works well in sauces, spreads,
dips, salad dressings, and in recipes that call for ricotta cheese.

Firm or Extra Firm Tofu

Firm and extra firm tofu have a curdled texture and hold their shape
well. They are best used in salads, scrambled tofu, stir-fry, and for grilling
and marinating.

Silken Tofu: Soft

Silken tofu contains more water and has a very smooth and delicate texture. Soft silken tofu works well in blended fruit shakes, soups, puddings,
and sauces.

Silken Tofu: Firm

Firm silken tofu works well in dishes that call for crumbled, steamed, or
cubed tofu.

Silken Tofu: Extra Firm

Extra firm silken tofu works well in stir-fry, or marinated and grilled, or
any other recipe that requires the tofu hold shape well.

TIPS ON PASTA

Pasta has really come into its own. Today there is a plethora of fresh and dry pastas in almost any shape you can imagine, found in most supermarkets. Some companies are now adding spinach, tomato, and herbs to their pasta. There are even pasta stores now where the only thing sold is fresh pasta.

It doesn't matter where you buy your pasta. The only thing you need to do is be sure that it has no egg in the ingredients. Although less common today, pasta makers in the past often added egg to their product. Occasionally, you will find a brand of fresh pasta that still contains egg.

Be sure to try some of the new pastas made with corn, rice, and quinoa. (See Resources). This is a great way to add variety to your pasta dishes.

As you begin incorporating vegetables into your meals, you will undoubtedly find that there are wonderful ways to combine vegetables. The chart above offers some suggestions.

Also, the cooking times for grains and legumes vary, as does the amount of water required, so be sure to check the charts that follow for the right combinations of water and time.

COMBINATIONS FOR ENJOYING VEGETABLES	
Corn and pimientos	Carrots and green beans
Cauliflower and green peas	Brussels sprouts and celery
Pearl onions, mushrooms, and green peas	Summer squash, tomatoes, and onions
Carrot slices and lima beans	Lima beans and corn
Mushrooms and green peas	Green cabbage, onions, and green bell pepper
Diced carrots and green beans	Brussels sprouts and carrot slices
Tomatoes, onions, and zucchini	Broccoli and cauliflower florets
Carrots, cabbage, and celery	Corn and peas
Celery and mushrooms	Eggplant, zucchini, onions, and tomatoes
Okra, onions, and tomatoes	

BEAN	COOKING TIMES FOR LEGUMES		
	Water	Cooking Time	Yield (cups)
ADZUKI BEANS (1/2 CUP)	2 cups	40 minutes	1 1/2
BLACK BEANS (1 CUP)	4 cups	2 hours	2
BLACK-EYED PEAS (1/2 CUP)	2 cups	1 hour	1 1/2
CHICK PEAS (1/2 CUP)	2 cups	1 hour	1 1/2
FAVA BEANS (1/2 CUP)	2 cups	40 minutes	1
GREAT NORTHERN BEANS (1/2 CUP)	2 cups	1 hour	1 1/2
KIDNEY BEANS (1/2 CUP)	2 cups	1 hour	1 1/2
LENTILS (1/2 CUP)	1 1/2 cups	40 minutes	1 1/2
LIMA BEANS (1 CUP)	2 cups	1 1/2 hours	1 1/4
MUNG BEANS (1 CUP)	2 1/2 cups	1 1/2 hours	2
NAVY BEANS (1 CUP)	3 cups	2 1/2 hours	2
PINTO BEANS (1/2 CUP)	2 cups	1 hour	1 1/2
RED BEANS (1 CUP)	3 cups	3 hours	2
SOYBEANS (1/2 CUP)	2 cups	2 hours, 20 min.	1 1/2
SPLIT PEAS (1/2 CUP)	2 cups	30 minutes	1

BAKING AND COOKING TIPS

Cooking Legumes

For best results, legumes, with the exception of lentils and peas, should soak for up to eight hours to assure that they cook evenly. Prior to soaking, be sure to rinse the legumes and inspect them for small stones. After the eight–hour soak, the water used should be poured out and fresh water added before cooking them. Doing so will reduce the tendency of legumes to produce intestinal gas. An option is to "quick–soak" legumes. This entails placing the legumes in water (3 cups for each cup of legumes), bringing to a boil, reducing heat, allowing to simmer for about three minutes, then removing from heat and letting stand covered for one hour. Drain the water, and start with fresh water before cooking.

Cooking Grains

When cooking grains it is best to use a smaller pot so that you do not loose much moisture in evaporation. When the liquid is added, the contents should fill half to three-quarters of the pot.

An option is to cook your grains in a slow cooker. A slow cooker takes about 8 hours to cook grains, but can be very convenient since it can work overnight while you sleep or while you are out during the day.

COOKING TIMES FOR GRAINS			
GRAIN (1 CUP)	Liquid	Method	Yield (cups)
BARLEY, PEARL	3 cups	Bring liquid to a boil. Add barley, stir and cover. Cook over low heat until water is absorbed and grain is tender, about 45 minutes.	3
BUCKWHEAT GROATS, ROASTED (KASHA)	1 1/2 cups	Bring liquid to a boil. Add groats, stir and cover. Cook over low heat 8 minutes. Remove from heat and let stand 5 minutes.	3
BULGUR BULGUR IS CRACKED WHEAT MADE FROM BERRIES THAT ARE STEAMED, THEN DRIED BEFORE CRACKING.	1 1/2 cups	(for pilaf): Bring liquid to a boil. Add bulgur, stir and cover. Cook over low heat 10 minutes. Remove from heat and let stand 10 minutes. (for salad): Bring liquid to a boil. Pour over bulgur. Let stand 5 minutes. Drain. Wrap in several thicknesses of cheesecloth and squeeze dry. Fluff with a fork.	2 1/2 1 3/4
COUSCOUS	1 cup	Bring liquid to boil. Add couscous, stir and cover. Remove from heat and let stand 10 minutes. Fluff with a fork.	2 3/4
MILLET	2 cups	Bring liquid to a boil. Add millet, stir and cover. Cook over low heat 10 minutes. Remove from heat and let stand 10 minutes.	3 1/2
OATS, ROLLED	2 1/2 cups	Bring liquid to a boil. Add oats while stirring. Simmer uncovered for 10 minutes.	2
POLENTA (COARSE CORNMEAL)	4 cups	Bring liquid to a boil. Add polenta gradually, whisking constantly. Cook over low heat, stirring often, until thick and creamy, about 20 minutes.	3 1/2
QUINOA	1 1/2 cups	Rinse quinoa well. Bring liquid to a boil. Add quinoa, stir and cover. Cook over low heat 15 minutes. Remove from heat and let stand 5 minutes.	2 1/2
RICE, BROWN	2	Bring liquid to a boil. Add rice, stir and cover. Cook over low heat 45 minutes. Remove from heat and let stand 5 minutes.	3 (long-grain); 2 1/2 (short-grain)
RICE, LONG-GRAIN WHITE (BASMATI TYPE; NOT CONVERTED RICE)	1 1/2 cups	Bring liquid to a boil. Add rice, stir and cover. Cook over low heat 18 minutes. Remove from heat and let stand 5 minutes.	3
RICE, SHORT-GRAIN WHITE	1 1/2 cups	Rinse rice in a sieve until water runs clear. Drain. Bring liquid to a boil. Add rice, stir and cover. Cook over low heat 25 minutes. Remove from heat and let stand 5 minutes.	2 3/4
RICE, WILD	2 1/2 cups	Bring liquid to a boil. Add rice, stir and cover. Cook over low heat 1 hour.	3

Replacing Eggs/Milk/Cream

Whether you are an avid cook or just have a few favorite recipes you like to prepare, there are some important tips you may wish to know about as you make the transition to more healthful eating.

Many of the recipes that call for eggs can be remedied by simply replacing egg with tofu. Pureed tofu (blended in a food processor or blender) can act as a replacement in recipes that call not only for eggs but for sour cream and yogurt. For example, one 12-ounce box of tofu will puree into 1-1/2 cups of "replacer." In recipes, 5 tablespoons of pureed tofu replace one egg.

Tofu, as well as soy and rice milks, also works well as a replacement in soup, gravy, sauce, dressing, dip, and spreads, and even mashed potato recipes that normally call for milk or cream.

Eggs that act as a "binder" in recipes can also be replaced using mashed potatoes or quick-cooking rolled oats. Another popular egg replacer is called Ener-G Egg Replacer. Made from potato starch, flour, and leavening, this powder mix is good to have on hand.

Finally, you may also wish to experiment with flaxseeds. Flaxseeds blended with water (1 tablespoon seeds with 1/4 cup water for each egg required) make a nutritious and flavorful egg replacer.

Replacing Meat

To replace meat in recipes for chili, stir–frys, and spaghetti sauce, use tempeh (made from fermented soybeans), texturized vegetable protein (TVP- made from compressed soy flour), or seitan (made from wheat protein). Tempeh and seitan are found in the refrigeration section of health food markets, and TVP is found with dry goods.

CHAPTER TWENTY-TWO

Recipes and Menus

In this chapter you will find the suggested menus and recipes for the first two weeks of your new way of eating. Depending on your personal tastes you may wish to mix and match the dishes differently. Feel free to do so. Although not specified in the recipes, it is assumed that organic ingredients will be used whenever possible. The second-best option is to use fruits, vegetables, herbs and other foods that have been locally grown. Your local farmers' market is a good source for both organic and locally grown foods.

Each dish listed on the daily menus will be followed by a page number where you will find the corresponding recipe. The exception is for dishes like oatmeal, the simple recipe for which can be found on any oatmeal box, cold cereals, tomato salsa and other condiments, fruit salad, and a few dessert items which are derived from a pre-mix that you can buy in your local natural foods market.

In pasta dishes, you are welcome to substitute alternatives such as quinoa pasta, corn pasta, brown rice pasta, or fresh whole wheat pasta. Either of these will work fine in the recipes. Note: while most dry pastas are fine, whole wheat pasta is best if it is purchased fresh, rather than dry. Seek out a local pasta shop for fresh whole wheat and other pasta variations.

Certain name brand products are suggested often because the products are available organic and or because the products have been tested and found to be the best choice from what is available. All name brands that have been recommended should be easily found in most natural foods markets and better health food stores. As an example, various Long Life Teas are recommended with the menus. Long Life is the only brand tea that could be found that states that they do not use a chlorine bleaching process on their tea bags (therefore their tea bags are dioxin-free), nor do they use staples to attach the tea bag string. Many Long Life teas are made with organic ingredients, and, frankly, they are delicious.

In some menus fresh vegetable juice is recommended. In many stores you can buy such juices prepared daily, but it is recommended that you make your own juice. This way, they will be even fresher, and you and the earth will not have the burden of more plastic with which to contend. A good juicer is an inexpensive and wise investment in your health.

Finally, although it is certainly not a requirement, it is recommended that you invest in quality cookware. Increasing attention has been focused on the health hazard of cooking with aluminum cookware, and most of what is on the market is aluminum. The reason is that aluminum is an excellent conductor of heat. However, it seems that the aluminum also has a tendency to be absorbed by food and ends up accumulating in the body. It is believed that there is strong relationship between aluminum accumulated in the brain and the onset of Alzheimer's and perhaps even Parkinson's disease. If you do choose to invest in cookware, we recommend two brands: Calphalon Teflon coated, or All-Clad stainless steel. Calphalon makes aluminum pans, so be sure to ask about their Teflon coated professional pan series. These pans will be a cinch to clean and will require no "greasing."

All-Clad uses an aluminum core for heat conductivity, and then coats the pan with an additional layer of stainless steel. This process protects your health, enhances cookware performance, and eliminates the chance of the cookware reacting with natural acids in food and thereby adversely affecting flavors. Either of these brands of cookware is available at most department stores.

DAY ONE

Breakfast
Blueberry Almond Pancakes (p. 242)
Cantaloupe or Honey Dew Melon
Long Life Early Morning Riser Tea

Lunch
Green Salad with Honey Dijon Dressing (p. 249)
Black Bean and Kale Soup (p. 244)
Barbara's Baked Corn Chips
Tomato Salsa
Pear Slices

Dinner
Caesar Salad with Homemade Croutons (p. 248)
Whole Wheat Pasta with Rich Mushroom Sauce (p. 266)
Warm Peach Crisp (p. 276)
Long Life Chamomile Tea

DAY TWO

Breakfast

Southwestern Tofu Scramble (p. 243)
Refried Beans
Warm Corn Tortillas
Salsa
Long Life Three Ginseng Tea

Lunch

Wild Rice Salad (p. 253)
White Bean and Broccoli Soup (p. 247)
Sour Dough Baguette or Pita Bread
Peach Slices and Blueberries
Carrot Juice

Dinner

Summer Vegetable Salad (p. 253)
Sweet Potato Pancake with Braised Greens
Lundberg's Elegant Rice Pudding
Long Life Cranberry Tea

DAY THREE

Breakfast

Hot Oatmeal with Apple Slices and Cinnamon
Raisin Bran Muffins (p. 243)
Banana
Long Life Echinacea & Goldenseal Tea

Lunch

Green Salad
Baked Potato with Tomato Salsa
Tofu Sour Cream
Steamed Broccoli
Sliced Watermelon
Mineral Water or Fresh Pressed Carrot Juice

Dinner

Arugula Salad with Tomato Vinaigrette Dressing (p. 253)
Grilled Yam Polenta with Lentil Sauce (p. 259)
Whole Grain Roll
Caramelized Pear Strudel (p. 273)
Long Life Tran-Kwil Tea

DAY FOUR

Breakfast

Cream of Wheat with Nutmeg and Sliced Bananas
Whole Wheat Toast
Cascadian Farms Organic Fruit Spread
Long Life Cranberry Tea

Lunch

Butternut Squash Wrap (p. 258)
Wild Rice or Quinoa
Tomato Salsa
Mineral Water

Dinner

Caesar Salad with Homemade Croutons (p. 248)
Whole Wheat Pizza with Roasted Peppers and Eggplant
Soymage Soy Parmesan Cheese Topping
Tapioca
Long Life Organic Peppermint Tea

DAY FIVE

Breakfast
Nature's Path Mesa Sunrise Cereal
(Corn, Flax & Amaranth)
Soy Milk or Rice Dream
Grapefruit
Long Life St. John's Wort Blend Tea

Lunch
Wild Rice Salad (p. 253)
Coleslaw (p. 254)
Steamed Broccoli
Barbecue Tofu Sandwich
Sliced Pear
Mineral Water

Dinner
Roasted Beet and Persimmon Salad (p. 250)
Barley Mushroom Risotto (p. 255)
Steamed Artichoke
Toasted Whole Wheat Pita Bread
Strawberry Cookie Bars (p. 275)
Long Life Detox Tea

DAY SIX

Breakfast

Blueberry and Almond Pancakes (p. 242)
Sliced Bananas and Strawberries
Long Life Ming Dynasty Tea

Lunch

Potato Salad with Flax Seeds (p. 250)
Black Bean and Kale Soup (p. 244)
Baked Corn Chips
Rye or Sourdough Bread
Red Flame Grapes
Mineral Water

Dinner

Green Salad with Honey Dijon Dressing (p. 249)
Tofu Stew with Yams (p. 269)
Quinoa or Brown Basmati Rice
Caramelized Pear Strudel (p. 273)
Long Life Organic Green Tea with Lemongrass

DAY SEVEN

Breakfast

Lundberg's Hot and Creamy Rice Cereal
(Amber Grain or Sweet Almond)
Whole Wheat Bagel
Cascadian Farms Organic Fruit Spread
Fresh Mango and Strawberries

Lunch

Summer Vegetable Salad (p. 253)
Lentil Soup with Yams and Lemon (p. 246)
Steamed Kale with Fresh Lemon
Whole Wheat Focaccia Bread
Mineral Water

Dinner

Spinach Cucumber Salad (p. 252)
Saffron Pilaf with Almonds and Peas (p. 264)
Steamed Brussel Sprouts
Mango Guacamole (p. 274)
Long Life Cranberry Tea

DAY EIGHT

Breakfast
Raisin Bran Muffins (p. 243)
Cream of Wheat Cereal with Apple Slices
Long Life Wellness for Women Tea
Cantaloupe

Lunch
Mediterranean Bean Salad (p. 249)
Curried Sweet Potato Soup (p. 245)
Raspberries and Blueberries
Pacific Bakery Spelt Bread, Toasted
Mineral Water

Dinner
Potato Salad with Flax Seeds (p. 250)
Boca Burger with Trimmings
(Tomato, Lettuce, Onions, etc.)
Follow Your Heart's Vegenaise Spread
Corn on the Cob
Whole Wheat Bun
Cascadian Farms Organic Fruit Sorbet
Long Life Echinacea & Goldenseal Tea

DAY NINE

Breakfast

White Wave Soy Yogurt
Nature's Path Organic Corn Flakes
Rice Milk or Soy Milk
Sliced Gala Apple

Lunch

Lentil Soup with Yams and Lemon (p. 246)
Roasted Vegetable Sandwich (p. 263)
Fresh Kiwi and Banana
Herbal Tea or Mineral Water

Dinner

Polenta Lasagna with Roasted Vegetables (p. 260)
Steamed Artichoke
Whole Wheat Bread
Warm Peach Crisp (p. 276)
Long Life Wellness for Women Tea

DAY TEN

Breakfast

Baked Mochi with Apple Sauce
Arrowhead Mills Bits O Barley Hot Cereal
Soy Milk
Blackberries and Peach Slices
Long Life Early Morning Riser Tea

Lunch

Broiled Portabello with Arugula (p. 256)
Whole Wheat Pita Bread, Toasted
Papaya and Cherries
Carrot-Beet Juice

Dinner

Stuffed Tomato with Lentils and Spinach (p. 267)
Steamed Lundberg Black Indonesian Rice
Warm Peach Crisp (p. 276)
Long Life Organic Chamomile Tea

DAY ELEVEN

Breakfast
Southwestern Tofu Scramble (p. 243)
Tomato Salsa
Warm Corn Tortillas
Sliced Mango
Long Life Cranberry Tea

Lunch
Caesar Salad with Homemade Croutons (p. 248)
White Bean Soup with Broccoli (p. 247)
Pacific Bakery Kamut Bread, Toasted
Fresh Pressed Carrot Juice or Mineral Water

Dinner
Roasted Eggplant Salad with Tofu and Ginger (p. 251)
Brown Rice Pasta with Provincial Sauce (p. 257)
Whole Grain Bread
Cascadian Farms Organic Fruit Sorbet
Long Life Sweet Elderberry Tea

DAY TWELVE

Breakfast

Hot Oatmeal with Blueberries and Banana Slices
Soy Milk or Rice Dream
Whole Grain Toast
Cascadian Farms Organic Fruit Spread
Long Life Three Ginseng Tea

Lunch

Spinach and Cucumber Salad (p. 252)
Barley with Lentil Sauce (p. 259)
Steamed Broccoli
Sliced Pear
Fresh Pressed Carrot-Celery Juice or Mineral Water

Dinner

Romaine Lettuce with Creamy Tofu Chive Dressing (p. 248)
Polenta Lasagna (p. 260)
Steamed Brussel Sprouts
Sourdough Baguette
Strawberry Cookie Bars (p. 275)
Long Life Digest Tea

DAY THIRTEEN

Breakfast

Nature's Path Heritage Muesli
Soy Milk or Rice Dream
Whole Grain Toast
Eden Organic Apple Butter
Sliced Pineapple and Guava
Long Life Wellness for Women Tea

Lunch

Spinach Cucumber Salad (p. 252)
Saffron Pilaf with Almonds and Peas (p. 264)
Sliced Apple
Mineral Water

Dinner

Butter Lettuce with Creamy Tofu Chive Dressing (p. 248)
Cooked Barley with Rich Mushroom Sauce (p. 266)
Steamed Broccoli
Strawberry Cookie Bars (p. 275)
Long Life Vanilla Spice Tea

DAY FOURTEEN

Breakfast

Nature's Path Mesa Sunrise Cereal
(Corn, Flax & Amaranth)
Soy Milk or Rice Dream
Raisin Bran Muffins (p. 243)
Blackberries and Pear Slices
Long Life Three Ginseng Tea

Lunch

Green Salad with Honey Dijon Dressing (p. 249)
Whole Wheat Spinach Lasagna (p. 272)
Fresh Peas
Whole Grain Bread
Sliced Banana
Mineral Water

Dinner

Roasted Eggplant Salad with Tofu and Ginger
Brown Rice Pasta with Muir Glenn Organic Garden Vegetable Sauce
Whole Grain Bread
Lundberg Elegant Rice Pudding
Long Life Wellness for Women Tea

THANKSGIVING DINNER

Roasted Beets and Persimmon Salad (p. 250)

Glazed Yams (p. 258)

Pumpkin Stuffed with Braised Vegetables (p. 262)

Wild Rice Salad (p. 253)

Chestnut Dressing (p. 265)

Steamed Green Beans

Quinoa with Rich Mushroom Sauce (p. 266)

Cranberry Relish

Whole Grain Roll

Caramelized Pear Strudel (p. 273)

Martinelli's Sparkling Apple Cider

4TH OF JULY PICNIC

Potato Salad with Flaxseeds (p. 250)

Coleslaw (p. 254)

Green Salad

Boca Burgers with Garnishes
(Tomato, lettuce, onion, pickle, ketchup, mustard)

Corn on the Cob

Grilled Peaches* with Vanilla Rice Dream
or Soy Ice Cream

*If you are grilling your Boca Burgers keep the grill hot for peaches.
Simply cut peaches in half, remove the pit and then cut into quarters.
Lay them skin-up on hot grill for 2-3 minutes. Remove from grill and
serve with Rice Dream or soy "ice cream".

SUNDAY BRUNCH

Southwestern Tofu Scramble (p. 243)

Tomato Salsa

Assortment of :
Raisin Bran Muffins (p. 243)
Baked Cinnamon Mochi
Warm Corn Tortillas

White Wave Soy Yogurt

Fresh Fruit Salad

Fresh Pressed Carrot, Apple, and Orange Juices

BLUEBERRY ALMOND PANCAKES
Yield: 4 servings

2 Tbs. flax seeds

2 Tbs. brown sugar

1 1/2 cups soy milk

1/2 tsp. vanilla extract

1 cup all purpose flour

1/4 cup wheat bran

1/4 cup oatmeal

2 Tbs. wheat germ

2 tsp. baking powder

1/2 tsp. baking soda

1 cup blueberry fresh or frozen

4 Tbs. sliced almonds

Blend flax seeds, brown sugar, soy milk and vanilla extract in a bowl. Mix in flour, wheat bran, oatmeal, wheat germ, baking powder and baking soda until smooth, then add blueberries. Spray a non-stick skillet with canola oil and place over medium heat. Pour 1/4 cup batter onto hot skillet. Cook until bottom is golden brown or spatula slips underneath pancake with ease. Sprinkle with almonds, flip, and cook remaining side.

Serve with jam or pure maple syrup.

RAISIN BRAN MUFFINS
Yield: 12 muffins

1/2 cup oat bran	2 oz. flax seeds
1/2 cup wheat bran	3/4 cup soft tofu
1 cup unbleached all-purpose flour	1/3 cup unsweetened applesauce
	3 oz. Sucanat or brown sugar,
1 1/2 tsp. baking soda	1/4 tsp. cinnamon
1 tsp. baking powder	1/8 tsp. lemon zest
1/2 tsp. salt	1/2 cup raisins

Preheat oven to 400 F. Spray a standard muffin pan lightly with canola oil.

In a medium bowl, combine brans, flour, baking soda, baking powder and salt. Stir to blend well.

In another bowl, combine flax seeds, tofu, applesauce, Sucanat or brown sugar, cinnamon, lemon zest and raisins. Whisk until smooth and well-blended. Add to dry ingredients and stir with a spoon just until batter is blended; do not overmix.

Spoon about 1/4 cup batter into each muffin cup, almost filling the cup. Bake for about 15 minutes or until the muffins spring back when touched. Let rest in pan for 5 minutes before removing.

SOUTHWESTERN TOFU SCRAMBLE
Yield: 4 servings

olive oil spray	1 pinch cumin
1/2 cup onions, peeled, diced 1/4-inch	3 Tbs. soy sauce
	1 tsp. turmeric
2 cloves garlic, chopped	1 tomato, diced 1/4-inch
1/4 cup seeded, diced green chili pepper or bell pepper	salt and pepper to taste
	1 Tbs. cilantro, chopped
1 lb. firm tofu, crumbled	garnish (cilantro, salsa)

Lightly spray a large non-stick saucepan with olive oil. Heat over medium heat. Add onions, garlic, and pepper. Cook while stirring until translucent. Mix crumbled tofu and seasonings and add to sautéed ingredients with tomato. Mix with wooden spoon. Season with salt and pepper to taste. Sprinkle with cilantro. Serve hot with salsa.

BLACK BEAN AND KALE SOUP
Yields: 8 servings

3 stems lemongrass, branch removed

4 cups vegetable stock

canola oil spray

3 cloves garlic chopped

1 small yellow onion diced

2 cups baking potatoes, peeled, cut in 1/2 -inch cubes

2 cups of cooked black beans (navy), homemade or canned with juice

1 tsp. cumin powder

1 bunch kale, stem removed and minced

1 tbs. lemon zest (organic)

2 tbs. lemon juice

1/2 cup tomato salsa

1/4 tsp. salt

1/4 pepper

Chop or crush 3 stems of lemongrass. Bring 4 cups of cold vegetable stock with the lemongrass to a boil and remove from heat. Cover and let infuse for twenty minutes. Preheat a medium saucepan sprayed with canola oil; sauté the onion and garlic until translucent. Add the potatoes and the infused vegetable stock and bring to a simmer for 15 minutes. Add the cooked beans and cumin powder and cook for 20 minutes or until the potatoes are soft. Add minced kale, cook for five minutes, then stir in lemon juice and lemon zest. Season with salt and pepper, garnish with tomato salsa.

CURRIED SWEET POTATO SOUP
Yield: 4 servings

canola oil spray
1/2 cup onions diced 1/2-inch
1 cup leeks, white part only,
   diced 1/2-inch
4 cups sweet potato, peeled
   and diced 1-inch
2 tsp. curry powder or 1/2 tsp.
   curry paste

5 cups vegetable stock
1 cup corn roasted
   (1 large ear of corn)
salt and pepper to taste
garnish with parsley or
   fresh cilantro

Preheat a medium saucepan sprayed with canola oil. Sauté the onion and leeks until translucent, without browning. Combine the sweet potato, curry powder, and vegetable stock in another large pot. Bring to a boil, reduce heat, and simmer for 30 minutes. Pour the mixture into a blender or food processor and blend until very smooth. Add roasted corn. (To roast the corn peel corn and roast whole in a preheated oven at 450 degrees or in broiler for 15 minutes, or until golden brown. Remove kernels with a knife). Reheat and season with salt and pepper. Garnish with parsley or fresh cilantro.

LEEK AND CUCUMBER SOUP
Yield: 4 or 5 servings

olive oil spray
1/2 cup yellow onion peeled,
     diced 1/2"
1/2 cup white leeks, diced 1/2"
1 cup potatoes, peeled,
     diced 1/2"
4 cups vegetable stock
4 cups (3 whole) cucumbers,
     peeled, seeded, diced to 1/4"

1 1/2 tsp fresh dill, chopped
salt and pepper
4 Tbs. firm tofu, diced 1/4 inches
     to garnish (optional)
1 tomato peeled, seeded
     and diced.

Preheat a medium saucepan sprayed with olive oil; sauté the onion and leek until translucent. Add the potatoes, vegetable stock and 3 cups of the cucumber, bring to a simmer for 30 minutes. Pour into a blender and puree until smooth. Return to saucepan and add remaining 1 cup cucumber and simmer for 5 minutes. Add dill and season to taste with salt and pepper. Garnish with diced tofu and tomato.

LENTIL SOUP WITH YAMS AND LEMON
Yield: 8 servings

olive oil spray
1 tsp. cumin seeds
1 onion, peeled and diced
     1/4-inch
1 celery stalk, diced 1/4-inch
1 carrot, peeled and diced
     1/4-inch
2 teaspoons chopped garlic
1 cup lentils

5 cups vegetable stock
3/4 cup yams, peeled and diced
     1/4-inch
1 cup diced tomatoes
1 tsp. coriander powder
4 Tbs. cilantro, chopped
juice of 1 lemon
zest of 1/4 lemon
salt (optional) and black pepper

Preheat a medium saucepan sprayed with olive oil. Add cumin seeds and cook until lightly brown. Add onions, celery, carrots, and garlic and sauté until translucent. Add lentils, vegetable stock, yams, tomatoes, and simmer for 30 minutes. Add coriander and simmer for another 10 minutes. Season with chopped cilantro, lemon juice, lemon zest, salt and pepper.

WHITE BEAN AND BROCCOLI SOUP

Yields: 4 servings

olive oil spray
3 cloves garlic chopped
1 small yellow onion diced
1 cup baking potatoes, peeled,
    cut in 1/2 -inch cubes
3 cups vegetable stock
4 cups cooked white (navy)
    beans, homemade or canned
    with juice

1 cup of broccoli florets
teaspoon lemon zest
2 tbs. lemon juice
1/2 cup diced tomato
salt and pepper to taste

Preheat a medium saucepan sprayed with olive oil. Saute the onion and garlic until translucent. Add the potatoes and vegetable stock and bring to a simmer for 15 minutes. Add the cooked beans and cook for 20 minutes or until the potatoes are soft. Add the broccoli florets and cook for five minutes. Stir in lemon juice, zest. Season with salt and pepper, garnish with diced tomato.

CAESAR SALAD WITH HOMEMADE CROUTONS
Yield: 3 cups

1 large head romaine lettuce, chopped into bite-size pieces, washed and dried

Croutons:

1 cup of bread cut in 3/8-inch dice

Caesar Dressing:

1/2 cup silken tofu or soft tofu

2 Tbs. grated Parmesan-style Soymage (soy cheese)

1/8 tsp horseradish

1 Tbs honey

1 Tbs. lemon juice

1 Tbs. red wine vinegar

2 tsp. Dijon mustard

1 garlic clove, degermed, minced

salt and black pepper to taste

For the croutons: Preheat oven to 375 F. Put diced bread on a baking sheet and bake until golden brown, about 10 minutes.

For the Dressing: Put all ingredients in a blender or food processor and blend until smooth. Season to taste.

To assemble salad, put romaine in a salad bowl. Add 1 cup croutons and dressing to coat leaves evenly. Toss well. Serve immediately.

CREAMY TOFU CHIVE DRESSING

1/2 cup soft tofu

2 tsp. Dijon mustard

2 Tbs. red wine vinegar

1/8 tsp. horseradish

1 Tbs. honey

2 Tbs. chopped fresh chives or green onions

1/2 tsp. black pepper

salt to taste (optional)

Put all ingredients in a blender or food processor and blend until smooth. Season to taste. If dressing is too thick, add water.

HONEY DIJON FLAX OIL DRESSING
Yield: 1 cup

1 tsp. honey	1/2 medium clove garlic
1/2 cup flax seed oil	1 Tbs. chopped chives
3 Tbs. red wine vinegar	3 Tbs. warm water
1 tsp. Dijon mustard	salt and pepper

Combine all ingredients except water and chives in a blender or food processor. Blend for 10 seconds. Add water and process an additional 10 seconds. Add chives and season to taste. Cover well and refrigerate for up to 5 days.

MEDITERRANEAN BEAN SALAD
Yield: 4 servings

1 medium cucumber, peeled, seeded and diced	1 Tbs. red wine vinegar
1/2 cup tomato (peeled optional) seeded and diced	1/2 Tbs. lemon juice
	1/2 medium clove garlic chopped
1 (15 oz.) can kidney beans, drained and rinsed	1 Tbs. chopped parsley
1/4 cup diced red onion	2 Tbs chopped mint
2 Tbs flax seed oil	salt and pepper to taste

Peel cucumber, halve it lengthwise, and scrape out seeds with a small spoon. Cut cucumber into 1/4-inch dice (you should have about 1 cup). Cut tomato in halves, remove seeds. In a medium bowl combine all ingredients and mix to blend. Season with salt and pepper. Garnish with fresh herbs.

POTATO SALAD WITH FLAX SEEDS
Yield: 8 servings

3 lbs. red-skinned potatoes
1 cup diced celery
1 cup diced red onion
1 1/2 tsp. salt
1/4 tsp. pepper

1/2 cup Honey Dijon Flax Oil
Dressing (p. 249)
1 Tbs. minced chives or
green onion
1 tsp flax seeds

In a steamer, steam the potatoes over boiling water, or boil in salted water covered, until tender when pierced, 30 to 40 minutes. When cool enough to handle, peel, then cut into 1/4 to 3/4 -inch dice.

In a large bowl, stir together potatoes, celery, onion, salt, and pepper. Add dressing and stir gently to combine. Taste and adjust seasoning with salt and pepper. Transfer to serving bowl and sprinkle with chives and flax seeds.

ROASTED BEET AND PERSIMMON SALAD
Yield: 4 to 8 servings

2 cups roasted beets, diced
(3 to 4 medium size pieces
per salad)
1 cup fuju persimmon, peeled
and sliced (2 medium size
pieces per salad)

1/4 cup green onions, minced
3 ounces honey Dijon dressing
(recipe follows)
2 cups of baby spinach
1/2 cup of pomegranate seeds
(optional)

Wash the beets. Wrap in aluminum foil or lightly spray with olive oil spray. Roast in a preheated oven at 375 degrees for 30 to 45 minutes or until vegetables are tender when pierced. When cool enough to handle, peel, and then cut into slices. Mince onion and slice persimmon. In a medium bowl combine beets, persimmon, onions and dressing and toss very gently. Serve immediately on a bed of spinach. Sprinkle pomegranate seeds on top.

ROASTED EGGPLANT SALAD WITH TOFU AND GINGER
Yield: 4 servings

1 eggplant
1/2 tsp. cumin seed
2 tsp. cilantro, chopped
4 oz. silken or soft tofu
1 1/2 Tbs. lemon juice
1/2 tsp. fresh ginger, peeled
and chopped finely

1 large tomato, peeled, seeded, diced
1 green chili (jalapeno) seeded, diced
1 clove garlic, chopped
salt and pepper to taste

Preheat oven to 375 degrees. Split the eggplant lengthwise. Brush each half with olive oil and season with cumin seeds, cilantro and salt and pepper. Place on a baking sheet cut side down and bake in a preheated oven at 375 degrees for 40 minutes or until very soft and lightly browned. Remove from oven and allow to cool. Scoop out the flesh with a spoon. Chop coarsely.

Blend tofu with lemon juice in a blender or food processor until smooth. In a medium bowl, combine all ingredients and season to taste. Note: Wear plastic gloves when working with jalapeno peppers — the oils can burn the skin and eyes.

SPINACH AND CUCUMBER SALAD
Yield: 4 servings

1 small cucumber peeled,
seeded and diced
1 cup chopped, cooked spinach,
fresh (see below) or frozen
1/2 cup tofu sour cream or
silken tofu.
1 clove garlic, green germ
removed, minced

2 Tbs. fresh mint, chopped
3 Tbs. lemon juice
1 tsp. lemon zest
1 tsp. Dijon mustard
1 tsp. cumin, ground
salt and pepper to taste

In a medium bowl, combine cucumber, spinach, tofu or tofu sour cream, garlic, mint, lemon juice, lemon zest and mustard. Mix well until smooth. Season to taste with cumin, salt and pepper.

To cook spinach:

Wash the spinach thoroughly. Drop the spinach leaves into a large amount of boiling salted (1 tsp. per quart) water. Mix, and let spinach boil, uncovered, for 1 minute. (If you are using frozen leaf spinach, defrost thoroughly, and separate the leaves.)

Immediately pour the entire contents of the pot into a colander or a sieve held over the kitchen sink. Add some ice cubes and let cold water run through for a minute to refresh the spinach—this will preserve its bright green color and also prevent any further cooking.

Squeeze as much water out of the spinach as possible before chopping.

SUMMER VEGETABLE SALAD

Yield: 4 to 6 servings

2 cup mixed greens
1/2 cup asparagus
1/2 cup fennel
1/2 cup carrots
1/2 cup zucchini

1/2 cup yellow zucchini
1/2 cup green beans
1 cup cooked chickpeas
1 cup tomato vinaigrette

Parboil vegetables in a large pot of boiling, lightly salted water. Cook vegetables in batches. Start with the vegetables that take longer to cook: fennel and carrots. Follow with the asparagus, green beans and the zucchini. Cook vegetables al dente (until just tender to the bite) and refresh in iced water to stop the cooking process and keep bright colors. Save water to use as a vegetable stock. Serve vegetables over greens and drizzle with tomato vinaigrette dressing.

TOMATO VINAIGRETTE DRESSING

4 Tbs. flax seed oil
1 cup tomato peeled seeded
    and diced
2 Tbs. red vine vinegar

1/2 medium clove garlic, germ
    removed, chopped
1 Tbs. parsley, chopped
1 Tbs. basil, chopped

Mix all ingredients in a bowl. Covered and refrigerated, dressing will keep for three days.

WILD RICE SALAD

Yield: 4 servings

2 cups cooked wild rice
1/2 Fuji or Golden apple,
    peeled, diced and cored
1/4 cup red onions, diced
    1/8-inch, soaked in cold water
1/2 cup corn, cooked

1/2 cup red bell peppers,
    diced 1/8-inch
1/4 cup green beans,
    blanched and cut 1/8-inch
1/4 cup peas, fresh cooked
    or frozen

Combine all ingredients in a bowl. Add dressing before serving, season with salt and pepper.

BARBECUE TOFU SANDWICH
Yield: 4 servings

1 (14 oz.) package firm tofu
  pressed
1 cup of Muir Glen organic
  barbecue sauce

2 cup of coleslaw
8 slices of wheat bread or
  4 Kaiser Rolls.

Slice tofu 3/4 inch thick; drain extra water. Marinate in barbecue sauce for 1 hour or more. Cook in a Teflon pan 5 minutes, until glazed (or grill, or broil). Serve with coleslaw in a sandwich using whole wheat bread or Kaiser Rolls.

COLESLAW
Yield: 4 servings (makes approx. 4 1/2 cups)

13 cups packaged shredded
  green and red cabbage or
  coleslaw mix
1 cup shredded carrot
3/4 cup soft tofu
1 tsp. horseradish
1 tsp. Dijon mustard

4 Tbs. sherry vinegar or
  white wine vinegar
1 1/2 Tbs. honey
1/4 tsp. celery seed
1 tsp. salt
1/4 tsp. black pepper

Combine tofu, horseradish, mustard, sherry vinegar, honey, celery seed, salt, and pepper in a blender or food processor and mix until smooth . Use 1/2 cup of dressing for 4 cups of coleslaw mix.

BARLEY, MUSHROOM, AND SOYBEAN RISOTTO
Yield: 4 servings

1 cups dried wild mushrooms
(Porcini, Morels,
or Chanterelles)
3 quarts vegetable stock, home
made (see recipe on page 260)
or store-bought
olive oil spray
3 tablespoons shallots, peeled
and finely chopped

1 garlic clove, minced
1 1/2 cups pearl barley
1 cup of fresh frozen soy beans
salt and pepper
2 tablespoons minced parsley
2 tablespoons minced chives
or green onion

Put mushrooms in a small bowl and cover with 2 cups hot water. Let soak 10 minutes. Remove mushrooms from water. Strain water to remove any dirt residue. Put the strained liquid in a saucepan with 3 quarts of vegetable stock and bring to a simmer.

Spray the bottom of a non-stick saucepan with olive oil spray. Heat pan over medium heat. Add shallots and garlic, stir until translucent. Add barley, wild mushrooms, and 5 cups boiling broth. Bring mixture to a simmer over moderately high heat, adjust heat to maintain a simmer, and cook 25 minutes, stirring occasionally. Add more hot broth, 1 cup at a time, stirring often and waiting until barley has absorbed most of the liquid before adding more. After 25 more minutes, the barley should be just tender. Add a little more liquid if barley seems underdone or mixture seems dry.

Risotto should be creamy, but not soupy. Season with salt and pepper. Remove from heat and stir in warmed soybeans. Garnish with parsley and chives. Serve immediately.

BROILED PORTABELLO WITH ARUGULA
Yield: 4 servings

olive oil spray
4 Portabello mushrooms caps,
    wiped
salt and pepper
1 clove garlic, minced

2 Tbs. balsamic vinegar
3 cups mesclun salad
1 cup arugula
2 Tbs. soy parmesan (Soymage)
1 cup Tomato Vinaigrette (p. 253)

Remove stems so mushroom are flat (save stems for soups or other recipes).

Spray Teflon pan with olive oil. Sprinkle the gills (black part of mushroom) with salt and pepper, and add garlic. Drizzle with balsamic vinegar. Heat pan and place mushrooms top down and cook on medium heat. Turn mushrooms using a plastic cooking utensil and sprinkle other side with salt, pepper, and garlic powder. (To broil, heat the broiler, lay the mushrooms on the broiler tray and spray with olive oil. Place the tray in the broiler about 1 1/2 inches from the heat. Broil until the mushrooms soften, about 4 minutes. Turn the mushrooms over to broil the other side until tender, about 3 minutes more.)

Distribute the mesclun and the arugula evenly on serving plates. Slice the mushroom into thin slices. Place slices on top. Spoon the vinaigrette evenly around the salad. Sprinkle with soy parmesan.

BROWN RICE PASTA WITH PROVENÇAL BASIL SAUCE
Yield: 4 Servings

1 cup julienned or shredded carrot
3/4 cup julienned or shredded green zucchini skin (optional)
3/4 cup julienned or shredded yellow zucchini skin or more green zucchini skin (optional)
1 1/2 cups vegetable broth
1/2 cup diced onion
1/4 cup diced celery
1/4 cup diced turnip
1/4 cup diced, peeled russet potato

1 can (15 oz.) small, white beans
1 cup tightly packed fresh basil leaves without flower (blanched optional)
4 cloves garlic
12 ounces brown-rice spaghetti or whole-wheat spaghetti
salt (optional)
1 cup broccoli florets
3/4 cup diced tomato
pepper
lemon wedges (optional)

Prep and cook time: About 50 minutes

Notes. Buy brown-rice pasta at a health food store or natural foods market (see Resources). Cut vegetables 5 to 6 inches long and the width of spaghetti with the julienne blade on an Asian shredder or mandolin, or, make long shreds with the wide tooth of a grater.

1. Cut carrot and the green and yellow zucchini skin, as described. (Save remaining zucchini for other uses.) Set aside.

2. In a 3- to 4-quart pan over high heat, bring broth, onion, celery, turnip, and potato to boiling. Reduce heat, cover, and simmer until potato is tender to bite, about 6 minutes. Add half the beans and their liquid; return to simmering, then cook, covered, for 5 to 10 minutes to blend flavors. Keep warm and set aside.

3. In a blender or food processor, blend remaining beans and liquid, basil, and garlic until smooth. Set aside.

4. Cook pasta, uncovered, in 4 quarts boiling water and 1 tablespoon salt until almost tender to bite, about 5 minutes; after 3 minutes, add broccoli. Stir in julienned vegetables and boil until just tender to bite, about 1 minute. Drain and rinse with hot water. Remove broccoli, and keep warm.

5. Stir basil mixture into broth mixture. Spoon into 4" wide, rimmed dinner plates. Mound pasta in the center. Scatter tomato and broccoli around plate rim. Offer pepper and lemon wedges.

BUTTERNUT SQUASH WRAP
Yield: 4 servings

1 teaspoon olive oil
1 tsp. cumin seed
1 clove of fresh garlic, minced
1/2 tsp. fresh ginger, peeled
   and chopped
1/2 cup onions, diced 1/2-inch
1/2 cup red bell pepper,
   seeded and diced 1/2-inch
1 cup yellow split peas
2 cups butternut squash, peeled,
   seeded, and diced 1/2 -inch
1 tsp. coriander, ground

2 tsp. curry
4 cups vegetable stock
1 Tbs. lemon juice
salt and pepper to taste
4 large whole-wheat flour
   tortillas
(lard- and hydrogenated oil-free)
1/4 cup mango chutney or
   sauce
tomato salsa
cooked rice

In a medium non-stick saucepan, add olive oil and lightly toast the cumin. Add garlic and ginger, stir, then and add onion, red bell pepper. Cook until translucent. Add split peas, butternut squash, curry, coriander and vegetable stock. Bring to a boil, reduce heat, cover and simmer for 45 minutes or until peas are thoroughly cooked. Add lemon juice. Season with salt and pepper. Serve in a wrap made with whole-wheat tortillas, basmati rice, tomato salsa, and mango sauce.

GLAZED YAMS WITH ORANGE AND CINNAMON
Yield: 8 servings

2 pounds yams or sweet potatoes,
   peeled and sliced 1/2-inch
1 cup orange juice
2 Tbs. pure maple syrup
2 Tbs. brown sugar

pinch of nutmeg
1/2 tsp. salt
1/4 tsp. black pepper
1/2 tsp. cinnamon

Arrange sliced yams, overlapped, in a baking pan. Mix the rest of ingredients and pour over yams. Cover and bake in a preheated oven at 375 degrees for 15 minutes. Uncover and continue to bake until liquid has reduced to a glaze and potatoes are tender, about 45 minutes.

GRILLED YAM POLENTA WITH LENTIL SAUCE
Yield: 8 servings

3 cups water
2 cups yams, peeled and grated
   or finely diced

1 1/2 cups polenta
2 tbs. fresh thyme leaves
salt and pepper to taste

In a large saucepan, combine the water and grated yams. Bring to a boil and simmer over medium-high heat for 15 minutes, or until the yams are falling apart. Mix with a whisk and stir in the polenta in a steady stream while whisking. Lower the heat. Stir with a spoon and cook until polenta is thick, about 10 minutes. Season with thyme leaves, salt and pepper.

Pour polenta into a baking pan lined with parchment paper and level surface to about 1-inch thick. Let cool and refrigerate for 1/2 hour or until firm. Unmold and cut into desired shape with a knife or cookie cutter. Grill on a preheated grill or non-stick pan.

Serve with lentil sauce below.

LENTIL SAUCE
Yield: 4 servings

1/2 onion, peeled, diced
   1/4-inch
1 green chili seeded, diced
   1/4 -inch
1 teaspoon finely chopped
   fresh ginger
1 clove garlic, chopped
1 Tbs. soy sauce
1/2 cup lentils
1 1/2 cups vegetable stock
   or water

1 cup tomatoes, peeled, diced
   and seeded 1/4-inch
1/2 tsp. cumin seeds, toasted
1/4 tsp. coriander powder
2 Tbs. cilantro, chopped
1/2 lemon (juice)
1 pinch lemon zest
salt (optional) and black pepper

Spray the bottom of a non-stick saucepan with olive oil. Heat pan over medium heat. Add onion, green chili, ginger and garlic and cook while stirring until translucent. Add the soy sauce. Add lentils, vegetable stock, and tomatoes and simmer for 30 minutes. Add toasted cumin and coriander and simmer another 10 minutes. Season with chopped cilantro, lemon juice, lemon zest, salt, and pepper.

PASTA PRIMAVERA WITH FRESH TOMATO

Yield: 6 servings

1 lb. soy penne pasta
1 cup green zucchini,
    sliced 1/4 inch
1 cup broccoli florets
1 cup red and/or yellow bell
    pepper, sliced 1/4 inch

1 small carrot, peeled and
    sliced 1/4 inch
1cup snow peas
1 ounce grated Soymage
    Parmesan cheese (optional)

Cook pasta in a large amount of boiling, salted water, or according to package directions; drain. Place in large serving bowl.

Steam vegetables al dente. Toss with pasta. Sprinkle with soy Parmesan and serve with fresh tomato sauce on top. Garnish with basil leaves.

FRESH TOMATO SAUCE

4 Tbs. flax seed oil
1 cup vine ripened tomato,
    peeled seeded and diced
1 Tbs. balsamic vinegar

1 medium clove garlic,
    degermed, chopped
4 Tbs. chopped basil

Mix all ingredients in a bowl. Covered and refrigerated, the sauce will keep for 3 days.

POLENTA LASAGNA WITH ROASTED VEGETABLES

Yield: 6 servings

4 cups water or vegetable broth
1 Tbs. rosemary

1 1/2 cups polenta
salt and pepper to taste

In a large saucepan, bring water to a boil. Sprinkle in the polenta in a steady stream while whisking. Lower the heat to medium. Stir and cook until polenta is thick, about 10 minutes. Add rosemary, season with salt and pepper. Pour polenta into a pan lined with parchment paper, smooth and level surface to cover two layers of about 8 by 12-inches. Let cool and refrigerate for 1 hour or until firm. Unmold and cut into desired shape to fit lasagna pan.

FILLING

Olive oil spray

1 eggplant

1 red onion, peeled and diced

1 large red bell pepper, seeded,
   cut in strips

4 garlic cloves, minced

2 cups mushrooms, diced

2 tablespoons minced
   fresh oregano

2 tablespoons minced fresh basil

1/2 cup cooked red beans or
   runner beans

1/4 cup grated soy Parmesan
   cheese (Soymage)

3 cups nonfat marinara sauce,
   homemade or store-bought

4 oz. grated soy mozzarella-style
   cheese (Soymage)

Split the eggplant lengthwise. Spray each half with olive oil and season with salt and pepper. Place on a baking sheet cut side down and bake in a preheated oven at 375 degrees for 40 minutes or until very soft and lightly browned. Let cool and scoop out the flesh with a spoon. Chop coarsely.

Preheat a medium nonstick saucepan, spray with olive oil then add red onion, red bell pepper and garlic. Cook while stirring until translucent. Add mushrooms. Stir and cook until liquid evaporates. Transfer to a large bowl and stir in roasted eggplant, oregano, basil, beans, and soy Parmesan. Spread 1-cup marinara sauce in bottom of a rectangular baking dish (approximately 8 x 12 inches). Top with a layer of polenta, then the filling (spreading it evenly), then another layer of polenta. Top with Soymage. Bake uncovered until hot throughout, about 30 minutes. Let stand 10 minutes before slicing.

PUMPKIN STUFFED WITH BRAISED VEGETABLES
Yield: 8 servings

1 large pumpkin, or two large
  kabocha squashes (4 1/2 to
  5 pounds each)
salt, pepper
cinnamon
olive oil spray
1 cup shallots peeled, halved
  (if large), or 2 cups peeled
  baby onions
6 garlic cloves, peeled and left
  whole, or, halved if large
1 cup diced turnips in large dice
2 cups carrots, in large dice,
  or 2 cups whole baby carrots
1/2 tsp. juniper berries, ground
1 cup wild mushroom (porcini
  or shiitake), caps only
2 cups butternut squash, peeled
  and diced 3/4-inch
1 Tbs. sugar

1/2 tsp. dried thyme
1 cup Vegetable Broth (p. 270)
  or store-bought

Garnishes (optional)
1 pound swiss chard, leaves only,
  parboiled for 6 minutes,
  refreshed and cut into small
  pieces
1 cups potato gnocchi (no fat
  added: cook gnocchi according
  to package and drain)
1 cup cooked beans
  (pinto, lima or runners)
1 cup frozen fresh soy beans
Suggested garnishes: roasted
  corn, beets, snowpeas, diced
  tofu, salt, pepper, ground
  cinnamon, dried juniper
  berries

Preheat oven to 350 degrees. Spray squash skin with olive oil. Bake squash whole about 45 minutes or until a knife can be easily inserted. (To prevent browning, cover with aluminum foil). Let stand 15 minutes, then cut a thick slice off the stem end to make a "lid." Remove seeds with a spoon. Season the cavities with salt, pepper and cinnamon. Set aside. If using acorn squash, use a half-squash per person. In a large non-stick saucepan, heat oil over medium heat. Add shallots, garlic cloves, turnips and carrots. Season with salt and pepper and juniper berries, and sauté for 4 to 5 minutes over medium heat. Add mushroom, butternut squash, sugar, and thyme. After 5 minutes, add vegetable broth. Bring to a boil and simmer uncovered, stirring often until liquid reduces to a glaze and vegetables are tender. Add garnishes (cooked Swiss chard, beans, potato gnocchi, soy beans). Fill the squashes with vegetable stew and serve.

ROASTED VEGETABLE SANDWICH
Yield: 4 servings

8 slices whole wheat foccacia or whole wheat bread
2 tomatoes, sliced
2 Tbs. basil leaves, cut in chiffonade
8 leaves lettuce (arugula)
4 Tbs. aioli sauce
Roasted vegetables
olive oil spray
2 japanese eggplants, roasted, peeled, chopped
1 cup shiitake mushrooms, quartered
1 zucchini sliced lengthwise, cut 1/4 inches
1 small red onion, sliced

Aioli Sauce
1/2 cup soft tofu
1 Tbs. whole seed mustard
1/2 tsp. lemon juice
1/2 tsp. red wine vinegar
1/2 tsp. chopped garlic, degermed
1/2 tsp. salt
1/4 tsp. black pepper, ground
1 pinch cayenne pepper
Mix all ingredients in a food processor

Split the eggplant lengthwise. Brush each half with olive oil and season with salt and pepper. Place on a non-stick baking pan, cut side down. Bake in a preheated oven at 375 degrees for 40 minutes or until very soft and lightly browned. Let cool and scoop out the flesh with a spoon. Chop coarsely.

Using a non-stick baking pan, arrange mushrooms, zucchini and red onions in single layer. Season with salt and pepper. Spray with olive oil and roast in preheated oven at 375 degrees for 15 minutes.

Spread Aioli on bread slices; arrange vegetables and garnishes on top and serve.

SAFFRON PILAF WITH ALMONDS AND PEAS
Yield: 4 servings

2 tsp. olive oil
1 tsp. cumin seed
1 cup diced onion
1/2 cup diced carrots
1/2 cup diced celery
1 cup long-grain rice, preferably,
    or instant brown rice
1/2 cup yellow or green
    split peas

1 tsp. coriander seeds, grounded
1 pinch saffron
2 oz. toasted almonds
3 cups vegetable stock or water
2 whole cloves
1/2 tsp. salt
1/4 tsp. pepper

In a large non-stick saucepan, heat oil over medium heat. Add cumin seed and toast lightly. Add onions, carrots, and celery and cook while stirring until soft and translucent. Add rice, split peas, coriander, saffron, almond, and vegetable stock and cloves. Season with salt and pepper. Bring to a boil. Cover, reduce heat to lowest setting, and simmer 25 minutes (for whole brown rice cook for 45 minutes). Let stand 5 minutes, covered. Transfer to a serving bowl and fluff with a fork. Remove the cloves before serving.

CHESTNUT DRESSING
Yield: 8 servings

2 tsp. canola oil
1 1/2 cups diced onion
1 cup diced green bell pepper
3/4 cup diced celery
2 cups quartered shitake caps
2 cups peeled diced apple
1/4 cup dried cherries
2 cups Vegetable Stock (p. 264)
2 cups roasted chestnuts, peeled
(or store-bought vacuum-
packed or canned),
roughly chopped

8 cups whole wheat or
sourdough bread,
in 1/2-inch cubes
4 Tbs. flax seeds
1/4 cup walnut chopped
1/2 cup minced parsley
1/2 tsp. dried thyme
1 Tbs. chopped fresh sage
1/2 tsp. salt
1/2 tsp. black pepper

Preheat oven to 375 degrees. Prepare a 9 by 12-inch baking dish nonstick. Lightly sprayed with canola oil.

In a large nonstick saucepan, heat oil over medium heat. Add onion, bell pepper, celery, and mushrooms. Saute over medium heat for 5 minutes until vegetables become soft. Add apple and dried Cherries.

Put bread cubes in a large bowl. Stir in vegetable broth, parsley, thyme, sage, salt, and pepper. Mix flax seeds with bread. Add sauteed vegetables and roasted chestnuts and mix well.

Put stuffing into prepared dish. Cover with aluminum foil and bake 20 minutes. Uncover and bake an additional 5 minutes to crisp the top.

WHOLE WHEAT PASTA WITH RICH MUSHROOM SAUCE
Yield: 4 servings

2 Boca Burger patties (2.5 oz. each) or vegetable burger
1 teaspoon olive oil
2 Tbs shallots or onions, peeled and diced
2 garlic cloves, minced
2 1/2 cups tomato sauce
3 cups fresh sliced cepes or shiitake mushrooms
1 tsp. fresh or 1/2 tsp. dried thyme
2 Tbs. chopped fresh basil
salt and pepper
1 pound dried whole wheat pasta (see Resources) or penne pasta

Grill or cook burgers according to package directions. Chop into 1/2-inch dice.

In a large non-stick saucepan, heat oil over medium heat. Add shallots and garlic and cook until soft. Add chopped burger, tomato sauce, mushrooms, and thyme. Bring to a simmer and cook 15 minutes, stirring occasionally. Stir in basil; season to taste with salt and pepper. Keep warm.

Bring a large pot of salted water to a boil over high heat. Add pasta and cook until al dente, according to package directions. Drain and transfer to a large warm bowl. Add sauce to coat. Serve immediately on warm plates.

Note: Whole Wheat pasta is best when purchased fresh from a pasta store.

STUFFED TOMATOES WITH LENTILS AND SPINACH

Yield: 6 servings

6 tomatoes
coarse salt
olive oil spray
1 cup chopped onions
1/2 cup chopped celery
1/2 cup chopped carrots
1 Tbs. minced garlic
3 cups vegetable stock

1 cup dried green lentils or
    brown
1 tsp. grounded coriander
2 bunches fresh spinach, washed
    and stemmed
2 tsp. olive oil
2 tsp. minced garlic

Preheat oven to 350 degrees. Cut the tops off the tomatoes, and, using a teaspoon, scoop out the pulp, leaving a 1/4 inch thick wall. Core the pulp and discard as many seeds as possible. Coarsely chop enough pulp to measure 1/2 cup. Set aside.

Sprinkle the tomato cavities with the coarse salt and place cut side down on paper for 30 minutes to drain.

Lightly spray the bottom of a large non-stick saucepan. Heat pan over medium heat. Add onions, celery, carrots and garlic, and cook while stirring until soft. Add the vegetable stock, lentils, coriander and the reserve tomato pulp. Bring to a boil. Reduce heat and simmer for 35 minutes, or until the lentils are just tender but not mushy. Set aside for 15 minutes.

To prepare spinach, heat 2 teaspoon olive oil in a non-stick sauté pan. Add the minced garlic. Add spinach and stir. Season with salt and pepper. Sauté until the leave are wilted but still bright green, 4 to 5 minutes. Drain extra water and cool.

Fill each hollowed-out tomato with the lentil stuffing and top with blanched spinach.

Bake covered at 350 degrees for 10 minutes, or until heated through.

Serve over grain such as brown rice, black rice, quinoa, wild rice, or millet.

SWEET POTATO PANCAKES WITH BRAISED GREENS
Yield: 4 servings

olive oil spray
2 cups peeled, grated potatoes
  (2 baking potatoes such
  as russet)
2 cups peeled, grated,
  sweet potato (2 yams)
2 Tbs. green onions
2 Tbs. unbleached flour
2 Tbs. Egg replacer

salt and pepper
1 pinch ground nutmeg
Garnishes
4 cups braising greens (spinach,
  bitter greens, mustard,
  baby red Swiss chard),
  stems removed
2 tsp. garlic, minced
1 Tbs. chopped chives

In a large bowl combine the potatoes, sweet potatoes, green onion, flour, egg replacer, salt, pepper, and nutmeg. Spray a large non-stick skillet lightly with olive oil. Set over moderate heat. When skillet is hot, drop about 1/3 cup mixture for each pancake. Flatten the pancake with a plastic spatula. Cook until golden-brown on both sides. Serve on a bed of braising greens. Garnish with chopped chives.

To prepare greens: Lightly spray the bottom of a large non-stick sauce pan with olive oil. Heat pan over medium heat. Add the minced garlic, stir, and add the greens. Season with salt and pepper. Add 2 Tbs. water. Sauté until the leaves are tender but still bright green, 4 to 5 minutes. Drain extra water before serving.

TOFU STEW WITH YAMS
Yield: 4 servings

olive oil spray
1/2 cup onions, cut 3/4 inches
1/2 cup chopped celery,
  3/4 inches
2 garlic cloves, peeled and sliced
1/2 cup diced red bell pepper
1 tsp. minced fresh ginger
1/2 cup mushrooms, shiitake or
  button quartered
1/2 cup turnips, diced 3/4 inches
1 cup yams, peeled diced
  3/4 inches
1/2 cup mirin (Japanese cooking
  wine or sweet sherry)

1 cup vegetable stock
1/4 cup soy sauce
1/2 cup sliced zucchini,
  1/4-inch
2 Tsp. fresh rosemary chopped
12 oz. firm tofu, pressed and
  cubed
Freshly ground black pepper
  to taste
salt to taste
cayenne
1 Tbs. cornstarch (optional)
Garnish:
1 green onion, chopped

Lightly spray a large non-stick saucepan with olive oil. Heat over medium heat. Add onions, celery, garlic, red bell pepper, and ginger, and sauté until soft and lightly colored. Add mushrooms, turnips, and yams. Add mirin and bring to a boil. Cook for two minutes to let alcohol evaporate, then add stock and soy sauce and bring to a boil. Reduce the heat and simmer for 15 minutes. Add the zucchini, rosemary and the tofu, and simmer 5 minutes. Season to taste with the pepper, cayenne, and salt. If stock is too liquid dissolve 1 tablespoon of cornstarch with 2 tablespoons of water. Add this to the stew while stirring, and simmer for one minute. Garnish with chopped green onions and serve over brown rice or pasta.

VEGETABLE STOCK
Yield: 8 servings

2 carrots, peeled, tops removed

2 cups mushrooms, sliced

2 yellow onions, peeled

1 leek, white part cut in half

6 celery ribs

1/2 bunch parsley stems

2 Tbs. coriander seeds

2 tsp. thyme

2 cloves garlic, halved

10 pepper corns

5 whole cloves

2 bay leaves

Wash all vegetables. Cut into 1/2-inch pieces. In a large pot add vegetables, cover with cold water, and bring to a boil. Simmer for 30 minutes. Turn off heat and let flavors infuse until cold. Strain.

This stock can be prepared in advance and either refrigerated for 3 to 4 days or frozen.

WHOLE WHEAT PIZZA WITH ROASTED PEPPERS AND EGGPLANT
Yield: 4 servings

olive oil spray

2 tsp olive oil

1 eggplant

2 cups shiitake mushrooms, sliced 1 red bell pepper cut into strips

1 Tbs. chopped garlic

1 cup red onion sliced

1 pizza dough recipe

2 cups canned tomato sauce

2 Tsp. chopped oregano or basil

2 oz. soy Parmesan or 4oz. mozzarella-style cheese (Soymage)

salt and pepper

Preheat oven to 375 degrees.

Split the eggplant lengthwise. Brush each half with olive oil and season with salt and pepper. Place on a lightly sprayed non-stick baking pan, cut side down. Bake in a preheated oven at 375 degrees for 40 minutes, or until very soft and lightly browned. Let cool and scoop out the flesh with a spoon. Chop coarsely.

Preheat a large nonstick baking pan. Add mushroom, bell pepper, garlic and red onions. Season with salt and pepper, spray with olive oil, and roast in preheated oven at 375 degrees for 15 minutes.

Dived dough into four equal pieces. Roll out each piece into round 1/4 inches thick. Spread with tomato sauce. Add vegetables, and top with parmesan, garlic, and herbs.

PIZZA DOUGH

1 1/2 cups organic whole wheat
    flour
1 1/2 cups organic, unbleached,
    all-purpose flour
1 pack, or 1 Tbs. dry, fast-rising
    yeast

1 1/4 cups warm water
1 tsp. chopped rosemary
1 tsp. honey
1/2 tsp. salt

In food processor, fitted with a metal blade, combine all-purpose flour, whole-wheat flour, honey, rosemary, fast-rising yeast and salt. Pulse to blend. With motor running, gradually add warm water through the feed tube. Keep machine running until dough forms a ball. Sprinkle with a little more flour if dough seems sticky. Transfer dough to a bowl, lightly spray with olive oil, and cover with plastic wrap. Allow dough to rise in a warm place for 30 minutes. Punch down, cover, and let rise again in a warm place until doubled, about 30 minutes.

To make dough by hand:

In a large mixing bowl, combine the yeast with 4tbs. flour and honey. Stir in the warm water and let the mixture stand until bubbly, about 10 minutes. Stir lightly. Add the salt and enough all purpose flour and whole wheat flour to make a dough that is soft and pliable, but not sticky. Lightly flour a large, flat work surface. Remove the from the bowl and knead on floured surface until it is smooth.

Transfer dough to a clean bowl, lightly spray with olive oil. Cover bowl with plastic wrap and allow dough to rise in a warm place for 30 minutes. Punch down, cover, and let rise again in a warm place until doubled, about 30 minutes.

WHOLE WHEAT SPINACH LASAGNA
Yield: 6 servings

2 tsp. olive oil
1/2 cup diced shallots
1 Tbs. minced garlic
2 cups diced mushrooms
1 package (10 oz.) frozen,
    chopped spinach, defrosted
    and drained
1 cup extra firm tofu, crumbled
1/4 cup polenta
1/4 cup flax seeds, ground
1/4 cup julienned fresh herbs
    (parsley,basil,oregano)

1/8 tsp. ground nutmeg
4 oz. Soy parmesan
salt and pepper
3 cups nonfat marinara sauce,
    homemade or store-bought
1 lb.fresh whole wheat lasagna
    or 1/2 lb. dried lasagna
    noodles
grated mozzarella-style cheese
    (Soymage)

Preheat oven to 400 degrees.

In a large non-stick saucepan, heat oil over medium heat. Add shallots and garlic and cook while stirring, until translucent. Add mushrooms. Stir and cook until liquid evaporates.

Put spinach in a large bowl and stir in crumbled tofu, polenta, flax seeds, fresh herbs, nutmeg, parmesan and the cooked mushroom mixture. Mix well and season with salt and pepper.

Cook lasagna in a large pot of boiling salted water until just tender. (Follow package directions for timing). Drain and refresh under cool water, pat dry. (If noodles are sticking, rinse briefly with cold water.) Spread 1-cup marinara sauce in bottom of a rectangular baking dish (approximately 8 x 12 inches). Top with a layer of noodles. Top with half the filling, spreading it evenly, then another layer of noodles. Top with remaining filling and a final layer of noodles. Spread marinara sauce evenly over the surface. Top with Soymage. Bake uncovered until hot throughout, about 25 minutes. If using fresh pasta, cut pasta to fit in baking dish and follow the same procedure as above, but bake for 45 minutes covered.

CARAMELIZED PEAR STRUDEL
Yield: Serves 4

8 Bartlett pears, peeled, cored
   and cut into 6 pieces
2 Tbs. brown sugar
2 Tbs. frozen apple juice
   concentrate
1 Tbs. lemon juice

1/2 tsp. organic lemon zest
1/2 tsp. cinnamon
3 to 4 (14" x 8") oil free phyllo
   sheets (whole wheat
   if possible)

Place pears, brown sugar, frozen apple juice concentrate and lemon juice in a Teflon pan, and cover with lid. Cook for 5 minutes. Remove lid so that liquids evaporate and stir until the pears caramelize. Remove pears, place them in a bowl, and season with cinnamon and lemon zest.

Lay 1 sheet of phyllo dough on a clean dry surface. Spray phyllo lightly with vegetable oil. Repeat procedure with 2 more phyllo sheets, stacking in layers.

Spread the pears in center, leaving a 11/2-inch border on each side, and roll sheet up lengthwise, turning in ends to enclose filling. Place roll on a baking sheet that has been sprayed with vegetable oil.

Bake in preheated oven (400 to 425 degrees) for approximately 20 minutes until golden brown. Serve with soy ice cream or Rice Dream (2 oz. per serving).

MANGO GUACAMOLE WITH BANANA CHIPS
Yield: 4 servings

1/4 cup tofu soft, pureed

2 cups ripe mango, peeled and
finely diced

2 Tbs. honey

1/2 tsp. fresh ginger, chopped
finely or grated

3/4 tsp. fresh mint leaves,
finely chopped

1/4 tsp. cinnamon powder

1/4 tsp. cardamon, ground

banana (optional) cut in
chips and toasted

Puree tofu in a blender until smooth or whisk in a bowl. Add remaining ingredients and mix. Serve with toasted banana chips (available from oriental or health food markets). You can make your own chips by slicing a banana lengthwise into very thin slices (use a mandoline). Put slices onto a baking sheet that has been lined with parchment paper and lightly sprayed with oil. Bake in a preheated oven at 375 for 25 minutes or until golden brown. Let cool, serve guacamole in a martini glass with chips.

STRAWBERRY COOKIE BARS
Yield: 20 bars

1 3/4 cups rolled oats
2 cups crisp brown rice cereal
3/4 cups whole wheat pastry
 flour
1/2 tsp. baking soda
2 Tbs. wheat germ
2 Tbs. flax seeds
1 cup honey
1 cup frozen white grape or
 orange juice concentrate
 (defrosted)

1 tsp. almond extract
1 tsp. vanilla extract
3/4 cup Shredded Wheat cereal,
 crushed
1 jar (10-oz.) fruit juice-
 sweetened Strawberry
 preserves

Preheat oven to 350 degrees.

In a large bowl, combine oats, brown rice cereal, flour, baking soda, wheat germ and flax seeds. Set aside.

In a bowl combine honey, juice concentrate, vanilla and almond extracts. Gently stir in cereal mixture.

In a baking dish, press 2 cups of cereal mixture in bottom of pan; reserve remaining cereal mixture.

In a small saucepan, melt preserves over medium-high heat, pour over cereal mixture and spread evenly. Top with reserved cereal mixture.

Bake at 350 degrees for 30 minutes, or until nicely browned. Cool and cut into bars.

WARM PEACH CRISP
Yield: 6 servings

Filling
1 Tbs. cornstarch
1 tsp. lemon juice
2 Tbs. peach jam
1 Tbs. plus 2 tsp. sugar
1 tsp. vanilla extract
1/2 tsp. cinnamon
4 cups peaches, peeled, pitted
   and sliced (about 6 medium
   peaches or 1 pound)

Crisp
2/3 cup rolled oats + 2 Tbs
   rolled oats
1/3 cup Grape-Nuts cereal
1 Tbs. peach jam

Preheat oven to 375 degrees. In a bowl, mix cornstarch, lemon juice, peach jam, sugar, vanilla and cinnamon. Add peaches and mix.

Make crisp topping: Combine 2/3 cup oats, Grape-Nuts, and jam in a food processor and process just enough to mix jam. Transfer to a bowl. Add 2 Tbs. rolled oats.

Transfer the peaches to a 9-inch pie pan. Spread the crisp topping evenly over the peaches. Bake until peaches are bubbly and topping is lightly browned, about 20 minutes.

EPILOGUE

Contrary to what most people believe, we are living at a most opportune time in terms of disease prevention. Today we know more about the causes of and ways to prevent not only cancers but numerous other chronic degenerative diseases, such as heart disease, hypertension, diabetes, and osteoporosis, than at any time in history. Yes, we are faced with more hazardous toxic chemicals in our lives than ever before, but we also have the knowledge of how we can navigate around those toxic chemicals so as to best protect ourselves from exposure. There is, however, a great disparity between what is well known in the scientific community and what reaches the general public. By and large, the public health organizations are still distributing pamphlets with dangerously dated information that contradicts much of what researchers have discovered in recent years. The gap is closing, however, slowly but surely, and we see more Americans empowered through this new knowledge, taking a proactive stance and protecting their health. Despite the dreadful cases we hear about most often, there are wonderfully uplifting cases to know about. One of my favorites is that of Ruth Heidrich, Ph.D. Diagnosed with breast cancer at age 47, she decided to take control of her life and do everything she could to influence her health. She made many of the lifestyle changes outlined in this book (vegan diet, regular exercise, etc.), and today, at the age of 63, she is healthy and thriving. Not only did she overcome her cancer, she also happens to be participating in and winning marathons, one after another. Her bone density is greater than the average 30-year-old American woman, in part because she avoids dairy products (she also doesn't take calcium supplements). Ruth is not an aberration; she is one of many women who have taken control of their lives and their health. She stands as a powerful icon to women the world over. The point is that you don't need to wait for a diagnosis to adopt the healthful principles outlined in this book. Be proactive; incorporate these principles into your life now, reap the many benefits, and know that you are fortifying your entire body to function at optimal health.

I know that as you adopt the principles herein, you are going to discover a whole new you, one that is energized, needs less sleep, is free from prior chronic pain, and is less likely to respond to stressful events in unhealthful ways. In general, you should experience a dramatic transformation that will support life-long wellness. Congratulations for seeking out this information. I wish you the very best of health!

Joseph Keon, Ph.D.

PART FOUR

Resources

"And as a truth I say unto you,
that there are three things which bring
the end of civilization,
even the mightiest that have ever been
and shall ever be...
impure air, impure water and impure food."

Zend Avesta 3000 BC

RECOMMENDED READING

Alternative Cancer Therapies

Goldberg, Burton; Diamond, John W.; Cowden, W. Lee, *Definitive Guide to Cancer* (Tiburon: Future Medicine Publishing, 1997).

Robbins, John, *Reclaiming Our Health* (Tiburon, CA: HJ Kramer, 1997).

Weed, Susun S., *Breast Cancer? Breast Health!*: The Wise Woman Way (Woodstock: Ash Tree Publishing, 1996).

Breast Cancer

Heidrich, Ph.D. Ruth, *A Race for Life* (Hawaii Health Publishers, 1415 Victoria St., #1106, Honolulu, HI 96822).

Kradjian, M.D., Robert M., *Save Yourself From Breast Cancer* (New York: Berkley Books, 1994).

Weed, Susun S., *Breast Cancer? Breast Health!*: The Wise Woman Way (Woodstock: Ash Tree Publishing, 1996).

Cookbooks

Johnson, Deborah Page, The Feel Good Food Guide: *Easy Recipes Free of Sugar, Wheat, Eggs, Yeast, Dairy and Soy!* (Naperville: New Page Productions, 1996).

Martin, Jeanne Marie, Vegan Delights: Gourmet Vegetarian Specialties (Madeira Park: Harbour Publishing, 1993).

McDougall, Mary, *The McDougall Plan Recipes, Volume One*, (New Winn Publishing, Inc., 1983).

Raymond, Jennifer, *The Peaceful Palate* (Heart & Soul Publications).

Saltzman, Joanne, *Amazing Grains: Creating Vegetarian Main Dishes with Whole Grains* (Tiburon: HJ Kramer, 1990).

Wasserman, Deborah, *Simply Vegan* (The Vegetarian Resource Group).

Endocrine-Disrupting Chemical Exposure

Colborn, Theo; Dumanoski, Dianne Meyers and John Peterson, *Our Stolen Future* (New York: Dutton, 1996).

Environmentalism

Hartmann, Thom, *The Last Hours of Ancient Sunlight* (Northfiled: Mythical Books, 1998).

Hawken, Paul, *The Ecology of Commerce* (New York: Harper, 1993).

Montague, Ph.D., Peter, editor, *Rachel's Environment & Health Weekly*
A weekly electronic health letter produced by the Environmental
Research Foundation, P.O. Box 5036, Annapolis, MD 21403; FAX (410)
263-8944; e-mail: erf@rachel.clark.net. This is an outstanding resource
covering issues of the environment and personal health. To subscribe,
send E-mail to rachel-weekly-request@world.std.com, with the single
word SUBSCRIBE in the message space. It's free.

Steingraber, Ph.D., Sandra, *Living Downstream: An Ecologist Looks at Cancer
and The Environment* (New York: Addison Wesley, 1997).

Hazards of Dairy Foods

Cohen, Robert, *Milk: The Deadly Poison* (Englewood Cliffs: Argus
Publishing, 1998).

Oski, Frank, M.D., *Don't Drink Your Milk* (New York: Health Services,
1983).

Hazards of Dry Cleaning

Rice, Bonnie and Jack Weinberg, *Dressed to Kill: The Dangers of Dry
Cleaning and the Case for Chlorine-Free Alternatives* (Greenpeace,
1994; (202)-462-1177).

Hazards of Meat

Lyman, Howard F., *Mad Cowboy: Plain Truth From the Cattle Rancher Who
Won't Eat Meat* (New York: Scribner, 1998).

Hazards of Medical Radiation

Beir, Committee on the Biological Effects of Ionizing Radiation, *Health
Effects of Exposure to Low Levels of Ionizing Radiation*, (National
Academy Press, 1990).

Gofman, M.D. John W., *Radiation-Induced Cancer* (San Francisco: CNR
Books, 1990).

Moss, Ralph W., *The Cancer Industry* (Brooklyn: Equinox Press, 1980).

Natural Hormone Therapy

Lee, M.D., John R., *What Your Doctor May Not Tell You About Menopause*
(New York: Warner Books, 1996).

Pesticide Education

Moses, M.D., Marion, *Designer Poisons*: How to protect your health and home from toxic pesticides. (San Francisco: The Pesticide Education Center, 1995).

Spirituality and Health

Dossey, Larry, M.D., *Prayer is Good Medicine* (San Francisco: Harper, 1996).

Dossey, Larry, M.D., and other contributors, *The Power of Meditation and Prayer* (Carlsbad: Hay House, Inc., 1997).

Stress Management

Eliot, Robert S. and Dennis L. Breo, *Is It Worth Dying For?: How To Make Stress Work for You—Not Against You* (New York: Bantam Books, 1984).

Hanh, Thich Nhat, *Peace Is Every Step: The Path of Mindfulness in Everyday Life* (New York: Bantam Books, 1991).

Kundtz, David, S.T.D., *Stopping: How To Be Still When You Have To Keep Going* (Berkeley, Conari Press, 1998).

Vegan Nutrition

Klaper, M.D., Michael, *Vegan Nutrition: Pure and Simple* (Hawaii: Gentle World, 1987); *Pregnancy, Children, and the Vegan Diet* (Hawaii: Gentle World, 1994).

Wellness

Barnard, Neal, M.D., *Food For Life* (New York: Crown, 1993).

Hitchcox, D.C., Lee, *Long Life Now* (Berkeley: Celestial Arts, 1996).

Justice, Blair, Ph.D., *Who Gets Sick* (Los Angeles: Jeremy P. Tarcher, 1987).

Keon, Ph.D., Joseph, *Whole Health: The Guide To Wellness of Body and Mind* (Mill Valley: Parissound, 1997).

McDougall, M.D., John, *The McDougall Plan* (Clinton: New Win Publishing, 1983).

Northrup, M.D., Christiane, *Women's Bodies, Women's Wisdom* (New York: Bantam Books, 1994).

Women's Wellness

Northrup, M.D., Christiane, *Women's Bodies, Women's Wisdom* (New York: Bantam Books, 1994).

MAGAZINES

Delicious!
1301 Spruce Street
Boulder, CO 80302
(302) 939-8440

Veggie Life
P.O. Box 57159
Boulder, CO 80322

Vegetarian Gourmet
P.O. Box 7641
Riverton, NJ 08077

Vegetarian Times
P.O. Box 570
Oak Park, IL 60303
(708) 848-8100

Organic Gardening
33 East Minore Street
Emmaus, PA 18098
(215) 967-8154

YES! A Journal of Positive Futures
PO Box 10818
Bainbridge Island, WA 98110
(206) 842-0216

E The Environmental Magazine
PO Box 2047
Marion, OH 43306
(815) 734-1242

Yoga Journal
2054 University Avenue
Berkeley, CA 94704
(510) 841-9200

ENVIRONMENTAL ORGANIZATIONS

Greenpeace
847 West Jackson Blvd.
Chicago, IL 60607
(312) 563-6060

World Wildlife Fund
(Can provide information about endocrine disrupting chemicals).
1-800-26-PANDA
Panda@wwfcanada.org

EarthSave
620-B Distillery Commons
Louisville, KY 40206
(502) 589-7676; internet: http://www.earthsave.org

Rainforest Action Network (RAN)
450 Sansome Street, Suite 700
San Francisco, CA 94111
(415) 398-4404

Earth Island Institute
300 Broadway, Suite 28
San Francisco, CA 94133
(415) 788-3666

Youth for Environmental Sanity (YES)
420 Bronco Road
Soquel, CA 95073
(831) 427-3646
http//:www.yesworld.org

PESTICIDE REFORM

Organic Trade Association
P.O. Box 1078, 20 Federal Street, #3
Greenfield, MA 01302
(413) 774-7511

Natural Organic Farmer's Association
411 Sheldon Road
Barre, MA 01005
(508) 355-2853

Pesticide Action Network, North America (PANNA)
49 Powell St., Ste. a500
San Francisco, CA 94102
(415) 981-1771
E-mail: panna@panna.org
http://www.panna.org

National Coalition Against the Misuse of Pesticides
701 East Street, SE
Washington, DC 20003
(202) 543-5450

Americans for Safe Food/ Center for Science in the Public Interest
1875 Connecticut Ave, NW
Washington, DC 20009-5728
(202) 332-9110

ORGANIC FOODS-MAIL ORDER / HOME DELIVERY

The following companies provide a variety of organic foods by mail order or through home delivery. If you have trouble finding organics in your neighborhood stores, contact one or more of these companies for a catalogue of their products.

Bay Area Organic Express
P.O. Box 460411
San Francisco, CA 94146
(415) 695-9688
(home delivery)

Blooming Prairie Warehouse, Inc.
2340 Heinze Road
Iowa City, IA 52240

Ecology Sound Farm
42126 Road 168
Orosi, CA 93647
(209) 528-3816

Mother's Organics
San Rafael, CA
(415) 454-2071
(home delivery)

Star Organic Produce, Inc.
P.O. Box 561502
Miami, FL 33256-1502
(305) 262-1242

Walnut Acres
Penns Creek, PA 17862
(800) 433-3998

The Organic Traveler's Guide to the Wine Country, 1998
Community Action Publications. An outstanding guide to northern California's wine country (including Mendocino, Sonoma and Napa Counties). Provides a directory of organic farms, restaurants, health food stores, wineries, catering, nurseries, herb stores, and related products and services. 36 pp. U.S. $4.50. Community Action Publications, 6984 McKinley Street, Suite 60, Sebastopol, CA 95472 (707) 829-2999; E-mail: PDines@compuserve.com

---

NON TOXIC PEST CONTROL

The Household Detective Primer: How to Protect Your Children from Toxics in the Home, 1998. The Children's Health Environmental Coalition (CHEC). Briefly describes hazards of common household products and presents basic information about how to avoid toxic chemicals such as pesticides in the home. Discusses non-toxic pest control alternatives for home and garden. 31 pp. U.S. $10. CHEC, PO. Box 846, Malibu, CA 90265; Phone (310) 573-9608; FAX (310) 573-9688; E-mail CHEC@checnet.org; web site: www.chec.org.

Grow Smart, Grow Safe: A Consumer Guide to Lawn and Garden Products (1998)

Reviews over 300 lawn and garden products, including pesticides, fertilizers, pest barriers, traps and related tools. Presents basic data about health and environmental effects, stressing least toxic and non-toxic pest management. Includes information about managing insect, slugs, snails, diseases, weeds and soil fertility. Contact: Washington Toxics Coalition, 4649 Sunnyside Ave. N., Suite 540 East, Seattle, WA 98103; phone (206) 632-1545; www.accessone.com/~watoxics/.

Reducing Your Risk From Pesticides (1998).

Presents basic fact sheet-style information about reducing pesticides risk by using alternatives to pesticides and finding ways to reduce pesticide exposure. Outlines recommendations for reducing pesticides in agriculture, urban environments and indoors. Contact: Kim Bilous, World Wildlife Fund, 90 Eglinton Ave E., Suite 504, Toronto, Ontario, M4P2Z7, Canada; phone (416) 489-4567, ext 261; email: kbilous@wwfcanada.org; web site: www.wwfcanada.org/reduce-risk/.

WATER PURIFICATION SYSTEMS

Multi-Pure Water Purification Systems
P.O. Box 4179
Chatsworth, CA 91313
(800) 622-9206

U.S. Pure Water Corporation
Greenbrae, CA
(800) 776-7654

Harmony/Seventh Generation
360 Interlocken Blvd., Suite 300
Broomfield, CO 80021
(800) 869-3446

National Sanitation Foundation
3475 Plymouth Road
PO Box 130140
Ann Arbor, MI 48105

(NSA certifies water filtration systems and can provide you with a list of certified brand filters)

BREAST SELF EXAM

Mammacare
930 N.W. 8th Ave.
Gainesville, FL 32601
(800) 626-2273

BREAST FEEDING

La Leche League International
9696 Minneapolis Ave
Franklin Park, IL 60131
(800) LA -LECHE

DIAGNOSTICS

Oncolab
Contact: Sam Bogoch, M.D., Ph.D.
36 The Fenway
Boston, MA 02215
(800) 922 8378
(Provides AMAS test discussed in Chapter 3)

American Academy of Thermology
2740 Chain Bridge Road
Vienna, VA 22181
(703) 938-6140
(For information about facilities using thermography)

La Clinique
Contact: Nancy Gardner-Heaven
712 D Street, Suite L
San Rafael, CA 94901
(415) 460-9722
Provides thermographic (radiation-free) diagnostic exams.

Therma-Scan, Inc.
Contact: Philip Hoekstra, Ph.D.
26711 Woodward Avenue, Suite 203
Huntington Woods, MI 48070
(248) 544-7276
Philip Hoekstra, Ph.D. works with holistically-oriented physicians in
interpreting diagnostic thermograms. Using thermography, Dr. Hoekstra
has personally screened more than 50,000 women since 1971.

WOMEN'S HEALTH/BREAST CARE/SUPPORT GROUPS

National Women's Health Network
1325 G Street NW
Washington, DC 20005
(202) 347-1140

National Breast Cancer Coalition
Washington, DC
(202) 296-7477

Bay Area Breast Cancer Network
4010 Moore Park Avenue
San Jose, CA 95117

Breast Cancer Action
Contact: Barbara Brenner
55 New Montgomery
San Francisco, CA
(415) 243-9301
bcaction@hooked.net

Breast Cancer Prevention Now
Contact: Polly Strand
P.O. Box 168
Gualala, CA 95445
(707) 884-1915

Cancer Prevention Coalition
520 North Michigan Avenue, Suite 410
Chicago, IL 60611
(312) 467-0600

National Women's Health Network
(202) 347-1140

Women's Environment and Development Organization
(212) 759-7982

American Menopause Foundation, Inc.
Madison Square Station
PO Box 2013
New York, NY 10010
(212) 475-3107

LEGAL ASSISTANCE

California Women's Law Center, Breast Cancer Legal Clinic
3460 Wilshire Blvd., Suite 1102
Los Angeles, CA 90010
(888) 774-5200
Provides legal (at no cost to low-income women) assistance with issues such as employment discrimination of survivors, insurance negotiation, housing, public benefits assistance, etc.

ALCOHOL CESSATION

Alcoholics Anonymous
World Services Office
P.O. Box 459 Grand Central Station
New York, NY 10163
(212) 870-3400

INTERNET SITES

Breast Cancer.Net
http://www.breastcancer.net/bcnmain.html

Community Breast Health Project (Stanford University)
http://www.med.stanford.edu:/CBHP

National Alliance of Breast Cancer Organizations
http://www.nabco.org

Oncolink-Breast Cancer Section
(University of Pennsylvania Cancer Center)
http://ww.oncolink.upenn.edu/disease/breast

The Susan G. Komen Foundation
http://www.breastcancerinfo.com

Y-Me National Breast Cancer Organization
http://www.y-me.org

PHYSICIAN ASSOCIATIONS

American Holistic Medical Association (AHMA)
4101 Lake Boone Trail, #201
Raleigh, NC 27607
(919) 787-5146

Physicians Committee for Responsible Medicine (PCRM)
5100 Wisconsin Avenue, Suite 404
Washington, DC 20016
(202) 686-2210

Physicians for Social Responsibility
1101 14th Street, NW, Suite 700
Washington, DC
(202) 898-0150

VEGETARIAN AND VEGAN SUPPORT GROUPS

Vegetarian and Vegan Support Associations
American Vegan Society
501 Old Harding Highway
Malaga, NJ 08328
(609) 694-2887

North American Vegetarian Society (NAVS)
P.O. Box 72
Dolgeville, NY 13329
(518) 568-7970

Vegetarian Nutrition Dietetic Practice Group
American Dietetic Association
216 W. Jackson Boulevard
Chicago, IL 60606
(312) 899-0040

Vegan Action
P.O. Box 4353
Berkeley, CA 94704
(510) 654-6297
http://www.Vegan.org

MIT Vegetarian Support Group
Massachusetts Institute of Technology
Cambridge, MA
http://www.mit.edu:8001/activities/vsg/home.html

Vegetarian Society of the United Kingdom
Parkdale, Dunham Road
Altrinchan, Cheshire
WA14 4QG England
(0161) 928-0793
Vegsoc@vegsoc.demon.co.uk.

Vegsource
http://www.vegsource.com

SUPPORT FOR EATING DISORDERS

Beyond Hunger, Inc.
Contact: Lauralee O. Roark
P.O. Box 151148
San Rafael, CA 94915
(415) 459-2270

MEDITATION / STRESS REDUCTION

Transcendental Meditation Center Directory
(800) 843-8332

Biofeedback Therapy Directory
Biofeedback Certification Institute of America
10200 West 44th Avenue, Suite 304
Wheat Ridge, CO 80033
(303) 420-2902

NON-TOXIC DRY CLEANERS ("WET CLEANERS")

For information about wet cleaners contact:
www.greenpeaceusa.org/campaigns/toxic/wetclean.html
or call the Center for Neighborhood Technology at
(773) 278-4800, ext 299 or visit their webpage at: http://www.cnt.org.

NON-TOXIC DENTISTRY

For general information about mercury-free dentistry and a directory of
dentists practicing mercury-free dentistry, contact:

Environmental Dentistry Association
(800) 388-8123

International Academy of Oral Medicine and Toxicology
P.O. Box 608010
Orlando, FL 32860-5831

HEALTH FOOD
STORES AND MARKETS

Alfalfa's, *Denver, Vail, CO*

Amigo Natural Grocery, *Taos, NM*

Bread and Circus, *MA*

Cornucopia, *Northhampton, MA*

Erewhon Market, *Los Angeles, CA*

First Alternative, *Corvallis, OR*

Food for Thought, *Westport, CT; Sebastopal, CA*

Fresh Fields *National*

Good Food Store, *Missoula, MT*

Healthy You Market, *Marco Island, FL*

Mrs. Gooch's, *Los Angeles, CA*

Oasis Natural Grocery, *Ithica, NY*

The Real Food Company, *Northern CA*

Super Natural Foods, *Corte Madera, CA*

The Vitamin Cottage, *Denver, CO*

Weaver Street Market, *Carrboro, NC*

Whole Foods Markets, *National*

Wild Oats Markets, *National*

Zucchini's, *Athens, GA*

RECOMMENDED ALTERNATIVE PRODUCTS

The products listed below are recommended because of their health benefits and because they are manufactured by socially and environmentally responsible companies helping to safeguard our personal and environmental health, and to conserve our vital natural resources. All of the listed products are available at Whole Foods Markets, Wild Oats Markets, and other fine health food stores, or by contacting the manufacturer directly using the phone numbers listed below.

TOFU

Morinaga Nutritional Foods, Inc.
2050 West 190th Street, Suite 110
Torrance, CA 90504
(800) 669-8638

Morinaga is the maker of Mori-Nu Tofu that is aeseptically packaged in shelf-stable, hermetically sealed containers that allows it to store unrefrigerated until opened.

NON-DAIRY BEVERAGES

Vitasoy USA
Brisbane, CA 94005
(800) VIT-ASOY
Soy milk available "light" and organic.

Edensoy
Eden Foods, Inc.
Clinton, MI 94236
Makers of soy milk available with beta carotene, and vitamins B_{12}, E, and D fortified.

Rice Dream
Imagine Foods, Inc.
350 Cambridge Ave, Suite 350
Palo Alto, CA 94306
Makers of rice milk available vitamin A, D, and calcium fortified.

Almond "Mylk"
Wholesome & Hearty Foods, Inc.
2422 S.E. Hawthorne Blvd.
Portland, OR 97214
(800) 636-0109
Almond milk beverage.

Westsoy
Westbrae Natural Foods
Carson, CA 90746
(310) 886-8200
Makers of organic calcium and vitamin A and D fortified soy milk.

PASTA SAUCES

Muir Glen
PO Box 1498
Sacramento, CA 95812
(916) 557-0900
Makers of organic pasta sauce, canned tomatoes, ketchup,
and barbecue sauce.

ALTERNATIVE PASTA

Rice Innovations, Inc.
PO Box 16
Pickering, Ontario
Canada L1V2R2
Makers of Pastariso brand rice pasta.

Quinoa Corp.
PO Box 1039
Torrance, CA 90505
Makers of Ancient Harvest brand quinoa pasta.

Purity Foods, Inc.
2874 W. Jolly Rd.
Okemos, MI 48864
Makers of Vita Spelt brand spelt pasta.

SPICES

The Spice Hunter
San Luis Obispo, CA 93401

Spice Garden
Modern Products, Inc.
PO Box 09398
Milwaukee, WI 53209
Makers of non-irradiated spices.

TEA

Long Life Herbal Teas
Randolph, NJ 07869
(973) 252-0233
Makers of organically grown herbal teas, free of caffeine and contained in non-bleached, dioxin-free tea bags, without staples.

BABY FOOD

Earth's Best
PO Box 887
Middlebury, VT 05753
(800) 442-4221
Makers of organic baby food.

Organic Baby
United Natural Foods, Inc.
Dayville, CT 06241
Makers of organic baby food.

Simply Pure
RFD 3, Box 99
Bangor, ME 04401
(800) IAM-PURE
Makers of organic baby food.

HOUSEHOLD PRODUCTS

Harmony/Seventh Generation
49 Hercules Drive
Colchester, VT 05446
(800) 869-3446

Makers of dioxin-free paper products (paper towels, facial tissues, tampons, cotton swabs, etc.), non-toxic household cleaning products (dish and laundry soap, window cleaner, etc.), non-toxic insect and pest deterrents, and water filtration systems.

Organic Cotton Alternatives
Organic Bedding and Accessories
(888) 645-4452

Earthlings
P.O. Box 659
Ojai, CA 93024
(888) GO-BABY-O
http://www.earthlings.net
Organic baby clothing and accessories.

ORGANIC CLOTHING

Wildrose Farm
http://uslink.net/~knierim
(218) 562-4864
Organic clothing and fabrics

Certified Jean Co.
Seattle, WA
(206) 286-9685
Organic denim jeans

BODY CARE/COSMETICS

Aubrey Organics
Tampa, FL 33614
(800) AUBREY H
Makers of non-toxic shampoos, conditioners, lotions
and other body care products.

Home Health Products, Inc.
949 Seahawk Circle
Virginia Beach, VA 23452
Makers of non-toxic body care products available in stores
and by mail order.

Organic Essentials
Organic Cotton Products
(800) 765-6491

HAIR COLOR

Light Mountain
Lotus Brands, Inc.
P.O. Box 325
Twin Lakes, WI 53181

Herbatint
Bioforce of America, Ltd.
Kinderhook, NY 12106

Naturcolor
Herbaceuticals, Inc.
Glen Ellen, CA 95442
Makers of non-toxic hair coloring.

To learn about other manufacturers who are working to make environmentally responsible and non-toxic products contact: Shopping for a Better World: Council on Economic Priorities (800)-729-4CEP; website: www.access pt.com/cep/ or contact The National Green Pages™ Co-op America (800) 58-GREEN, http://www.coopamerica.org

To learn about the source of toxic chemicals that are produced in your area, visit the Environmental Defense Funds' Scorecard website at: http://www.scorecard.org. Through a simple process of entering your zip code, this free service can provide you with a wealth of information, including the names of companies that are producing toxic waste in your area, what specific chemicals they manufacture and the types of health problems associated with such chemicals, and much more.

NOTES

1   Physicians Committee for Responsible Medicine, *Good Medicine* 2, Spring 1997, p. 17.
2   Miller, Barry A., et al., "Recent incidence trends for breast cancer in women and the rele-
    vance of early detection: An update," *CA —A Cancer Journal for Clinicians* 43 (1993):27-41.
3   *Marin Independent Journal*, July 14, 1997, A:1.
4   Proctor, Robert N., *Cancer Wars: How Politics Shapes What We Know and Don't Know About
    Cancer* (New York: Basic Books, 1995).
5   Muir, C.S., et al., "The world cancer burden: Prevent or perish," *British Medical Journal* 290
    (1985):5-6.
6   *The Surgeon General's Report on Health and Nutrition*, U.S. Department of Health and
    Human Services, DHHS (PHS) Publication No. 88-50210, 1988.
7   EarthSave Foundation, *Realities for the 90's* : Facts drawn from *Diet for a New America* by
    John Robbins. EarthSave Foundation, 600 Distillery Commons, Suite 200, Louisville, KY
    40206-1922; (800) 362-3648.
8   Henderson, H. E. et al., "Toward the primary prevention of cancer," *Science* 254
    (1991):1131-1138.
9   Herman, Marcia E., "Secondary sexual characteristics and mensus in young girls seen in
    office practice: A study from the Pediatric Research in Office Settings Network," *Pediatrics*
    99 (1997): 505-12.; Lee, Peter A., "Normal ages of pubertal events among American males
    and females," *Journal of Adolescent Health Care* 1 (1980) 26-29.
10 Kagawa, Y., "Impact of the Westernization of the nutrition of Japanese: Changes in
    physique, cancer, longevity and centenarians," *Preventive Medicine* 7 (1978):205-17.
11 Ibid.
12 *Newsweek* "The Bountiful Breast" June 1, 1998, p. 71.
13 Petralao, N I., et al., "Breast secretory activity in non-lactating women, postpartum involu-
    tion, and the epidemiology of breast cancer," *National Cancer Institute Monograph* 47
    (1977):161-64; Siskind, V., et al., "Breast cancer and breast feeding: Results from an
    Australian case-control study," *American Journal of Epidemiology* 130 (1989):229-36; Yoo, K.Y.,
    et al., "Independent protective effect of lactation against breast cancer in young women,"
    American Journal of Epidemiology 135 (1992):726-733.; Newcomb, P. A., et al., "Lactation and
    a reduced risk of premenopausal breast cancer," *New England Journal of Medicine* 330
    (1994):81-87.
14 *Newsweek* "The Bountiful Breast," June 1, 1998, p. 71.
15 Colditz, Graham A., et al., "The use of estrogens and progestins and the risk of breast can-
    cer in postmenopausal women," *New England Journal of Medicine* 332 (1995):1589-93.
16 Swanson, Christine, et al., "Alcohol consumption and breast cancer risk among women
    under age 45 years," *Epidemiology* 8 (1997):231-37; Rosenberg, L. et al., "Breast cancer and
    alcoholic beverage consumption," *Lancet* 1 (1982):267; Longnecker, Mathew, "Do hormones
    link alcohol with breast cancer?," 85 (1993):692-93; Ewertz, Marianne, "Alcohol consump-
    tion and breast cancer risk in Denmark," *Cancer Causes and Controls* 2 (1991): 247-52; Kato,
    I., et al., "Alcohol consumption in cancers of hormone related organs in females," *Japan
    Journal of Clinical Oncology* 19 (1989):202-7.
17 Reichman, Marsha, et al., *Journal of the National Cancer Institute* 85 (1993):722-27.
18 Longnecker, M. P., et al., "A meta-analysis of alcohol consumption in relation to risk of
    breast cancer," *Journal of the American Medical Association* 260 (1988):652-56.
19 Reichman, M. E., et al., "Effects of alcohol consumption on plasma and urinary hormone
    concentrations in premenopausal women," *Journal of the National Cancer Institute* 85
    (1993):722-27.

20   MacGregor, R. R., "Alcohol and immune defense," *Journal of the American Medical Association* 256 (1986):1474-79.

21   *U.S. News and World Report* "For Babies, Weight Could Spell Fate," May 5, 1997, pp. 75-76.

22   Ballard-Barbash, R., et al., "Body fat distribution and breast cancer in the Framingham study," *Journal of the National Cancer Institute*. 82 (1990):286-90.

23   Hankinson, Susan, *Journal of the American Medical Association* (JAMA) 278 (1997):1407.

24   Goodwin, Pamela, et al., "Body size and breast cancer prognosis: A critical review of the evidence," *Breast Cancer Research and Treatment* 16 (1990):205-14.

25   Zhang, Shumin, et al., "Better breast cancer survival for postmenopausal women who are less overweight and eat less fat," *Cancer* 76 (1995):275-83.

26   Davis, Devra Lee, et al., "Environmental influences on breast cancer risk," *Science & Medicine* May/June (1997):56-63; Morabia, Alfredo, et al., "Relation of breast cancer with passive and active exposure to tobacco smoke," *Journal of Epidemiology* 143 (1996): 918-28.

27   *San Francisco Chronicle*, January 6, 1998.

28   Paulsen, Paul, "The Cancer Business" *Mother Jones* (May/June 1994):41.

29   Frankl, S., et al., "Women: Decrease your health risks," *Total Health* December (1993):26.

30   Spratt, J.S., et al., "Geometry, growth rates and duration of cancer and carcinoma-in-situ of the breast before detection by screening," *Cancer Research* 46 (1986):970-74; Wright, C. J., et al., "Screening mammography and public health policy: The need for perspective," *The Lancet* 346 (1995):29-32.

31   Plotkin, D., "Good news and bad news about cancer," *The Atlantic Monthly* (June 1996):82.

32   Wright, C. J., et al., "Screening mammography and public health policy: The need for perspective," *The Lancet* 346 (1995):29-32.

33   Peterson, Norma, "Mammograms may rupture in situ cysts, causing invasive cancer," *Breast Cancer Action Newsletter* 38 (1996):9; Watmough, D. J., et al., "X-ray mammography and breast compression," *The Lancet* 340 (1992):122.

34   Shore, R. E., et al., "Breast neoplasms in women treated with x-rays for acute postpartum mastitis," *Journal of the National Cancer Institute* 59 (1977):813-22; Modan, B., et al., "Increased risk of breast cancer after low-dose radiation," *The Lancet* (1989):629-31.

35   Goffman, John, *Preventing Breast Cancer* (San Francisco: CNR Books Committee for Nuclear Responsibility, Inc., 1996); http://www.ratical.com/radiation/CNR).

36   Bassett, Lawrence, et al., "Mammography and breast cancer screening," *Surgical Clinics of North America* 70 (1990):775-95.; Davis, D. L., et al., "Mammographic screening," *Journal of the American Medical Association* 271 (1994):152-53.

37   Hull, Jennifer Bignham, *Wall Street Journal* Wednesday, December 11, 1985, Dow Jones & Company, Inc.

38   Logan-Young, W. W., et al., (letter-to-the-editor) *New England Journal of Medicine* 328 (1993):811.

39   *Newsweek*, "Beyond the Mammogram," February 24, 1997, p. 59.

40   Hoekstra, Philip, "Screening for breast cancer and heart disease," *Alternative Medicine Digest* 22 (1996) :36-42.

41   Abrams, Martin B., et al., "Early detection and monitoring of cancer with the anti-malignin antibody test," *Cancer Detection and Prevention* 18 (1994):65-78; Bogoch, S., et al., "In vitro production of the general transformation antibody related to survival in human cancer patients: Anti-malignin antibody," *Cancer Detection and Prevention* 12 (1988):313-20; Bogoch S., et al., "Malignin antibody and early malignancy," *The Lancet* 337 (1991):977.

42   Day, P. J., et al., "The diagnosis of breast cancer: A clinical and mammographic campari-son," *Med Journal Astral* 152 (1990):635-39.

43   Elwood, JM., et al., "The effectiveness of breast cancer screening in young women," *Current Clinical Trials* 2 (1993):227.

44 Howe, G. R., et al., "Dietary factors and risk of breast cancer: combined analysis of 12 case-control studies," *Journal of the National Cancer Institute* 82 (1990):561-69.

45 Tannenbaum, A., et al., "Nutrition in relation to cancer," *Advances in Cancer Research* 1 (1953):451-65.

46 Cohen, L. A., et al., "Dietary fat and mammary cancer. I. Promoting effect of dietary fats on N-nitrosomethylurea-induced rat mammary tumorigenesis," *Journal of the National Cancer Institute* 77 (1986):33-42; Jacobs, M.M., *Exercise, Calories, Fat, and Cancer* (New York: Plenum Press, 1996)

47 Greenwald, P., "The potential of dietary modification to prevent cancer," *Preventive Medicine* 25 (1996):41-43; Wynder E. L., et al., *Breast cancer: The Optimal Diet* (New York. Plenum Press, 1992), pp.143-53.

48 Wynder, E. L., et al., "Breast cancer: Weighing the evidence for a promoting role of dietary fat," *Journal of the National Cancer Institute* 89 (1997):766-75.

49 Committee on Diet, Nutrition and Cancer, *Diet, Nutrition and Cancer* (Washington, DC: National Academy Press, 1982).

50 Micozzi M. S., et al., *Macronutrients: Investigating Their Role in Cancer* (New York: Marcel Dekker, Inc., 1992).

51 Boyar, Andrea P., et al., "Recommendations for the prevention of chronic disease: The application for breast disease," *American Journal of Clinical Nutrition* 48 (1988):896-900.

52 Jacobs, M. M., *Exercise, Fat, and Cancer* (New York: Plenum Press, 1992), p. 147.

53 Buell P., "Changing incidence of breast cancer in Japanese-American women," *Journal of the National Cancer Institute* 51 (1973):1479-83; Kinlen, L., "Meat and fat consumption and cancer mortality: A study of strict religious orders in Britain," *Lancet* 42 (1982):946-49.

54 Decarli, A., et al., "Macronutrients, energy intake, and breast cancer risk," *Epidemiology* 8 (1997):425-28.

55 Hirayama, T., "Epidemiology of breast cancer with special reference to the role of diet," *Journal of Preventive Medicine* 7 (1972):173-74.

56 Toniolo, P., et al., "Consumption of meat, animal products, protein and fat and risk of breast cancer: A prospective cohort study in New York," *Epidemiology* 5 (1994):391.

57 Parkin, D. M., et al., "Cancer incidence in five continents," International Agency for Research on Cancer Lyon, France, Vol. IV (1992).

58 Wynder, E. L., et al., "Comparative epidemiology of cancers in the United States and Japan," *Preventive Medicine* 6 (1977):567-94.

59 Rose, D. P., et al., "International comparisons of mortality rates for cancer of the breast, ovary, prostate, and colon and per capita food consumption," *Cancer* 58 (1986):2363-71.

60 Kelsey, Jennifer L., et al., "Epidemiology and prevention of breast cancer," *Annual Reviews of Public Health* 17 (1996):47-67.

61 Thomas, David B., and Margaret K. Karagas, *Cancer Epidemiology and Prevention* (2nd Ed.) (New York: Oxford University Press, 1996):236-54.

62 Buell, P. "Changing incidence of breast cancer in Japanese-American women," *Journal of the National Cancer Institute*. 51 (1973):1479-83; Wynder, E. L., et al., "Comparative epidemiology of cancers in the United States and Japan: A second look," *Preventive Medicine* 67 (1991):746; Tominaga, S., "Cancer incidence in Japanese in Japan, Hawaii, and western United States," *National Cancer Institute* 69 (1985):93-98; King H., et al., "Patterns of site-specific displacement in cancer mortality among migrants: Chinese in the United States," *American Journal of Public Health* 75 (1985):237-42; Shimizu, H., et al., "Cancer of the prostate and breast among Japanese and white immigrants of Los Angeles county," *British Journal of Cancer* 63 (1991):963-66.

63 R. et al., "Dietary fat reduction and plasma estradiol concentration in healthy pre-menopausal women," *Journal of the National Cancer Institute* 77 (1990):129-34.

64   Heber, David, et al., "Reduction of serum estradiol in postmenopausal women given free access to low-fat high-carbohydrate diet," *Nutrition* 7 (1991):137-39; Wynder, E. L., "The dietary environment and cancer," *Journal of the American Dietetic Association* 71 (1977):385-92; Ingram D. M., et al., "Effect of a low fat diet on female sex hormone levels," *Journal of the National Cancer Institute* (1987); Prentice, R., et al., "Dietary fat reduction and plasma estradiol concentration of healthy postmenopausal women," *Journal of the National Cancer Institute* 82 (1990):129-34;

65   Goldin, Barry R., et al., "Effect of diet on the plasma levels, metabolism and excretion of estrogens," *American Journal of Clinical Nutrition* 48 (1988):787-90.

66   Newman, S. C., et al., "A study of the effect of weight and dietary fat on breast cancer survival time," *American Journal of Epidemiology* 123 (1986):767-74.

67   Zhang, Shumin, et al., "Better breast cancer survival for postmenopausal women who are less overweight and eat less fat," *Cancer* 76 (1995):275-83.

68   Gregorio, David, et al., "Dietary fat consumption and survival among women with breast cancer," *Journal of the National Cancer Institute* 75 (1985):37-41.

69   Nordevang, E., et al., "Dietary habits and mammographic patterns in patients with breast cancer," *Breast Cancer Research and Treatment* 26 (1993):207-15.

70   Byrne C., et al., "Mamographic features and breast cancer risk: Effects with time, age and menopause status," *Journal of the National Cancer Institute* 87 (1995):1622-29.

71   Ibid.

72   Boyd, N. F., et al., "The short-term effects of a low-fat, high carbohydrate diet on radiologic features of the breast," *Cancer Epidemiologic Biomarkers Prev* 37 (1996):269.

73   Davis, Devra Lee, et al., "Medical hypothesis: xenoestrogens as preventable causes of breast cancer," *Environmental Health Perspectives* 101 (1993):372-77; Flack, F. et al., "Pesticides and polychlorinated biphenyl residues in human breast lipids and their relationship to breast cancer," *Archives of Environmental Health* 47 (1992):143-46; Unger, M., et al., "Organochlorine compounds in human breast fat from deceased with and without breast cancer and in a biopsy material from newly diagnosed patients undergoing breast surgery," *Environmental Research* 34 (1984):24-28.

74   Mussalo-Rauhamaa, H., et al., "Occurrence of beta-hexachlorocyclohexane in breast cancer patients," *Cancer* 66 (1990):2124-28.

75   Rogan, Walter, et al., "Pollutants in breast milk," *New England Journal of Medicine* 302 (1980):1451; Laug, E. P. et al., "Occurrence of DDT in human milk," *Archives of Industrial Hygiene* 3 (1951):245-46; Edo, D. et al., "Purgeable organic compounds in mother's milk," *Bulletin of Environmental Contamination and Toxicology* 28 (1982):322-28.

76   Prenctice, Ross, et al., "Dietary fat and cancer: Consistency of the epidemiologic data, and disease prevention that may follow from a practical reduction in fat consumption," *Cancer Causes and Control* 1 (1990):81-97.

77   Cohen, L. A., et al., "Modulation of N-nitrosomine methylurea induced mammary tumor promotion by dietary fiber and fat," *Journal of the National Cancer Institute* 83 (1991):496.

78   Oski, Frank, *Don't Drink Your Milk* (New York: Health Services, 1983).

79   Oski, Frank A., "Is bovine milk a health hazard?," *Pediatrics* 75 (suppl) (1985):182-86; Oski, Frank *Don't Drink Your Milk* (New York: Health Services, 1983).

80   Parke, A., "Rheumatoid arthritis and food: A case study," *British Medical Journal* 282 (1981):2027.

81   Soothill, J. F., et al., "Is migraine food allergy? A double-blind controlled trial of oligoantigenic diet treatment," *The Lancet* October 15, (1983):865-69.; Monro, Jean, et al., "Food allergy in migraine: Study of dietary exclusion and RAST," *The Lancet* July 5, (1980): 1-5.

82   Parke, A., "Rheumatoid arthritis and food: A case study," *British Medical Journal* 282 (1981):2027.

83 Lucas, A., et al., "Breast milk and subsequent intelligence quotient in children born preterm," *Lancet* 339 (1992):261-64.

84 Coombs, R.S., et al., "Allergy and cot death: With special focus on allergic sensitivity to cow's milk and anaphylaxis," *Clinical and Experimental Allergy* July 20 (1990):359-66.

85 Jukka, Karjalainen, et al., "A bovine albumin peptide as a possible trigger of insulin-dependent diabetes mellitus," *New England Journal of Medicine* 30 (1992):302-7.

86 Willet, Walter, et al., "Galactose consumption and metabolism in relation to the risk of ovarian cancer," *Lancet* 7 (1989):66-71.; Cramer, D.W., et al., "Characteristics of women with a family history of ovarian cancer, galactose consumption and metabolism," *Cancer* 74 (1994):1309-17.

87 Feskanich, D., et al., "Milk, dietary calcium, and bone fractures in women," *American Journal of Public Health* 87 (1997):992-97; Recher, R., "The effect of milk supplements on calcium metabolism and calcium balance," *American Journal of Clinical Nutrition* 41 (1985):254.

88 Keon, Joseph, *Whole Health: The Guide to Wellness of Body and Mind* (Mill Valley: Parissound, 1997); Food and Drug Administration, Investigator's Report, *FDA Journal* 30 (1996):34.

89 Epstein, Samuel A., "Potential public health hazards of biosynthetic milk hormones," *International Journal of Health Services*, 20 (1990):73-84.

90 *Postgraduate Medicine* 95 (1994):113-20.

91 Outwater, J., et al., "Breast cancer and dairy product consumption," *Medical Hypothesis* 6 (1997):453-62.

92 Mettlin, C. J. et al., "A case-control study of milk-drinking and ovarian cancer," *American Journal of Epidemiology* 132 (1990):871-76; Mettlin, C.J., "Invited commentary: Progress in nutritional epidemiology of ovarian cancer," *American Journal of Epidemiology* 134 (1991):457-59.

93 Northrop, Christiana, *Women's Bodies, Women's Wisdom* (New York: Bantam Books, 1994).

94 Sternglass, E. J., et al., "Breast cancer: Evidence for a relation to fission products in the diet," *International Journal of Health Services* 23 (1993):783-804.

95 Jukka, Karjalainen, et al., "A bovine albumin peptide as a possible trigger of insulin-dependent diabetes mellitus," *New England Journal of Medicine* 30 (1992):302-7; Working Group on Cow's Milk Protein and Diabetes Mellitus, *American Academy of Pediatrics*, "Infant feeding practices and their possible relationship to the etiology of diabetes mellitus," *Pediatrics* 94 (1994):752-54.

96 Epstein, Samuel, "Potential public health hazards of biosynthetic milk hormones," *International Journal of Health Services* 20 (1990):73-84.

97 O'Conner, Amy, "BGH linked to cancer in humans," *Vegetarian Times*, March 1996, p.18.

98 Hankinson, Susan E., et al., "Circulating concentrations of insulin-like growth factor I and risk of breast cancer," *The Lancet* 351 (1998):1393-96; Peyrat, J. P., et al., "Plasma insulin-like growth factor-1 (IGF-1) concentrations in human breast cancer," *European Journal of Cancer* 29 (1993):492-97.

99 Steinman, David, *Diet for a Poisoned Planet* (New York: Ballentine, 1990).

100 Investigator's Report, *FDA Journal* 30 (1996):34.

101 "Virus-like particles in cow's milk from herd with a high incidence of lymphosarcoma," *Journal of the National Cancer Institute* 33 (1964):2055-64; Marie-Liesse, G., "Effects of brucellosis vaccination and dehorning on transmission of bovine leukemia virus in heifers on a California dairy," *Canadian Journal of Veterinarian Research* 54 (1990):184; Ferrer, J., "Milk of dairy cows frequently contains a leukemogenic virus," *Science* 213 (1981):1014., "Beware of the Cow" (editorial) *Lancet* 2 (1974):30., *British Medical Journal* 61 (1990):456-9., *British Journal of Cancer* 61 (1990):456-9; Olmstead, Mirsky M., et al., "The prevalence of proviral leukemia virus in peripheral blood mononuclear cells at two subclinical stages of infection," *Journal of Virology* 70 (1996):2178.

102   Feskanich, D., et al., "Milk, dietary calcium, and bone fractures in women: A 12-year prospective study," *American Journal of Public Health* 87 (1997)992-97.

103   Remer, T., et al., "Estimation of the renal net acid excretion by adults consuming diets containing variable amounts of protein," *American Journal of Clinical Nutrition* 59 (1994):1356-61.

104   Schulsinger, D., "Effect of dietary protein quality on development of aflatoxin B-induced hepatic prenoplastic lesions," *Journal of the National Cancer Institute* 81 (1989):1241-45.

105   Hitchcox, Lee, Long Life Now (Berkeley: Celestial Arts, 1996), p. 59.

106   Barnard, Neal D., et al., "Animal waste used as livestock feed: Dangers to human health," *Preventive Medicine* 26 (1997):1-4.

107   Hitchcox, Lee, *Long Life Now* (Berkeley: Celestial Arts, 1996), p. 59.

108   Bryan F. L., et al., "Health risks and consequences of Salmonella and Campylobacter jejuni in raw poultry," *Journal of Food Processing* 58 (1995):326-44.

109   *The New York Times*, "25 Million Pounds of Beef is Recalled," August 22, 1997, A:1.

110   Meeker-Lowry, Susan, *Meat monopolies: Dirty Meat and the False Promise of Irradiation* (Washington: Food & Water, Inc., 1996),p. 5.

111   Ibid.

112   Rashmi, Sinha, et al., *Cancer Research* 54 (1994):6154-59.

113   Jacobs, R.M., et al., "Detection of multiple retroviral infections in cattle and cross-reactivity of bovine immunodeficiency-like virus," *Canadian Journal of Veterinary Research* 56 (1992):353-59; Cockerell, G. L., et al., "Seroprevelance of bovine immunodeficiency-like virus and bovine leukemia virus in a dairy cattle herd," *Veterinary Microbiology* 31 (1992):109-16; *AIDS* 6 (1992):759., Actavirologica 34 (1990):19-26.

114   Schecter, Arnold, et al., "Congener-specific levels of dioxins and dibenzofurans in U.S. food and estimated daily dioxin toxic equivalent intake," *Environmental Health Perspectives* 102 (1994):962-66.

115   "Is your food safe?" CBS News, *48 Hours*, transcript (Burrelle's Information Services, New Jersey, March 2, 1994), 20-22.

116   *Time* "Something smells foul," 17 (October 1994):42.

117   Wempe, J. M., et al., "Prevalence of Campylobacter jejuni in two California chicken processing plants," *Applied Environmental Microbiology* 45 (1983):355-59.

118   *Rachel's Environmental Weekly*, #555, Environmental Research Foundation, P.O. Box 5036, Annapolis, MD 21403; (410) 263-8944.

119   Steinman, D., *Diet for a Poisoned Planet* (New York: Ballentine, 1992).

120   Clarkson, Thomas, "Environmental contaminants in the food chain," *American Journal of Clinical Nutrition* 61 (1995):682-86.

121   Ibid.

122   *Vegetarian Times* "Something Fishy," February 1996, p. 18.

123   Gibbs, Gary, *The Food That Would Last Forever* (New York: Avery, 1993)

124   *Federal Register*, December 3, 62 (1997):64112.

125   *San Francisco Chronicle* "New study on breast cancer, fats," January 12, 1998: A:4.

126   Kwiterovich, Peter O., "The effect of dietary fat, antioxidants, and pro-oxidants on blood lipids, lipoproteins, and atherosclerosis," *Journal of the American Dietetic Association* 97 (1997):S31-S41.

127   Erasmus, Udo, *Fats and Oils* (Burnaby, Canada: Alive Books, 1986), p. 111.

128   Ibid.

129   Willet, W. C., et al., "Intake of fatty acids and risk of coronary heart disease among women," *The Lancet* 341 (1993):581-85.

130   Kohlmeier, Lenore, et al., "Adipose tissue trans fatty acids and breast cancer in the European Community Multicenter Study on antioxidants, myocardial infarction, and breast cancer," 6 *Cancer Epidemiology, Biomarkers & Prevention* (1997):705-10.

131 United Nations Environment Program, *Industry and the Environment* UNEP Environment, no 7.

132 Nasca, P. C., et al., "Relationship of hair dye use, benign breast disease, and breast cancer," *Journal of the National Cancer Institute* 64 (1980):23-8; Shore, R.E., et al., "A case-control study of hair dye use and breast cancer," *Journal of the National Cancer Institute* 62 (1979):277-83; Kinlen, L. J., et al., "Use of hair dyes by patients with breast cancer: A case-control study," *British Medical Journal* 2 (1977):366-68.

133 "No-pest strip insecticide poses an unacceptably high risk of cancer in people and pets," *Journal of Pesticide Reform* (Spring 1988):29.

134 Colborn, Theo, Dumanoski, Dianne, and Peterson Myers, John, *Our Stolen Future* (New York: Dutton, 1996)

135 Soto, A.M., et al, "The pesticides endosulfan, toxaphene, and deildrin have estrogenic effects on human estrogen-sensitive cells," *Environmental Health Perspectives* 102 (1994):380-383.; sumpter, J.P., et al., "Vitellogenesis as a biomarker for estrogenic contmination of the aquatice enviroment," *Environmental Health Perspectives* 103 (Suppl) (1995):173-178.; Bergeron, J.M., et al., "PCBs as environmental estrogens: Turtle sex determination as a biomarker of environmental contamination,: *Environmental Health Perspectives* 102 (1994):780-781.

136 *Rachel's Environmental Weekly*, #555, Environmental Research Foundation.

137 Ibid, #390, 414.

138 European workshop on the impact of endocrine disruptors on human health and wildlife, December 2-4, 1996, Weybridge, U.K., Report of proceedings, European Environmental Agency, Kongens Nytorv 6, DK-1050, Copenhagen K, Denmark.

139 Thomas K, Colborn T. Organochlorine endocrine disruptors in human tissue. In: Chemically-induced alterations in sexual and functional development: the wildlife/human connection (Princeton, NJ: *Princeton Scientific Publishing*, 1992):365-394.

140 *Rachel's Environmental Weekly*, #555, Environmental Research Foundation.

141 As per note 136.

142 Steingraber, Sandra, *Living Downstream: An Ecologist Looks at Cancer and the Environment* (New York: Addison Wesley, 1997).

143 PVC Bulletin, Greenpeace.1436 U Street. Washinton, DC; 800-326-0959; http://www.green-peace.org/usa.

144 Howard, Phillip, et al., *Handbook of Environmental Fate and Exposure Data for Organic Chemicals: Solvents*, (Chelsea, MI: Lewis Publishers, 1990), pp. 418-29; Bonnie Rice and Jack Weinberg, *Dressed to Kill: The Dangers of Dry Cleaning and the Case for Chlorine-Free Alternatives*, (Chicago, IL: Greenpeace and Pollution Probe, 1994); to order call Greenpeace at (800) 326-0959.

145 Ott, Wayne R., et al., "Everyday exposure to toxic pollutants," *Scientific American*, February (1998):86-91.

146 Larson, David E., *Mayo Clinic Family Health Book* (New York: William Morrow and Company, 1990),p. 330.

147 as per note 144, (Greenpeace).

148 Howard, Phillip H., et al., *Handbook of Environmental Fate and Exposure Data for Organic Chemicals, Vol 2., Solvents* (Chelsea, MI: Lewis Publishers, 1990), pp 418-29.

149 U.S. Environmental Protection Agency, *Environmental News*, May 11, 1993.

150 *Delicious!* April 1995, 38.

151 Diamond, John W., et al., *Definitive Guide to Cancer* (Tiburon, CA: Future Medicine Publishing, 1997), p. 580.

152 Fox, Martin, *Healthy Water* (Portsmouth: Healthy Water Research, 1990), p. 12.

153 *Journal of the American Medical Association* (JAMA) 264 (1990):500-2; 266 (1991):513-14; 268 (1992):746-48; 273 (1995):775-76.

154   News Release from the National Federation of Federal Employees (NFFE) local 2050, July
       2, 1997, (this organization consists of toxicologists, chemists, biologists at the United States
       Environmental Protection Agency, Washington, DC contact: J. William Hirzy, Ph.D., Senior
       Vice President, NFFE; (202) 260-4683); LI, XS, et al., "Effects of fluoride exposure on intelli-
       gence in children," *Fluoride* 28 (1995):189-92.
155   Ibid.
156   Weininger, Jean, *San Francisco Chronicle*, October 6, F:1.
157   Wigle, D. T., et al., "Contaminants in drinking water and cancer in Canadian cities,"
       Canadian Journal of Public Health 77 (1986):335-41.
158   *USA Today*, February 18- 20 1994.
159   *The Mayo Clinic Family Health Book* (New York: William Morrow, and Co, 1990)p. 330.
160   Walter H. Corson, *The Global Ecology Handbook:* What You Can Do About the
       Environmental Crisis (Boston: Beacon Press, 1990), p. 252.
161   Steingraber, Sandra *Living Downstream* (New York: Addison Wesley, 1997)., Corliss, Julie,
       "Pesticide metabolite linked to breast cancer," *Journal of the National Cancer Institute* 85
       (1993):602-606.; Davis, Devra Lee, et al., "Medical Hypothesis: Xenoestrogens as pre-
       ventable causes of breast cancer," *Environmental Health Perspectives* 101 (1993):372-377.;
       "Environmental factors and breast cancer," *Journal of the National Cancer Institute* 85
       (1993):647.; Hunter, David J., et al., "Pesticide residues and breast cancer: The harvest of a
       silent spring?" *Journal of the National Cancer Institute* (85) (1993):598-599.; Wolf, Mary S., et
       al., "Blood levels of organochlorine residues and risk of breast cancer," *Journal of the
       National Cancer Institute* 85 (1993):648-652.; "Breast cancer may have link to Pollutants,"
       USA Today, Octover 15, 1993.; "Pesticides linked to leap in breast cancer," *Sacramento Bee*,
       August 9, 1993.; "Studies give pesticides role in breast cancer: Scientific evidence growing,
       Congress told," *Washington Post*, October 22, 1993.
162   Falck, F., et al., "Pesticides and polychlorinated biphenyl residues in human breast lipids
       and their relation to breast cancer," *Archives of Environmental Health* 47 (1992):143-46. Wolff,
       M.S., et al., "Blood levels of organochlorine residues and risk of breast cancer," *Journal of
       the National Cancer Institute* 85 (1993):648-652. Dewally, E., et al., "High organochlorine
       body burden in women with estrogen receptor positive breast cancer," *Journal of the
       National Cancer Institute* 86 (1994):232-234; Mussalo-Rayganaam, H., et al., "Occurrence of
       beta-hexachlorocy-clohexane in breast cancer patients," *Cancer* 66 (1990):2124-2148.
163   Pesticide Action Network (PANNA) *Pannups*, vol. 7, no. 2, June 1997.
164   Leibman, James. Pesticide Action Network *Rising Toxic Tide: Pesticide Use in California* 1991-
       1995 (San Francisco: PANNA, 1997).
165   Visitainer, M.A., et al., "Helplessness, chronic stress and tumor development,"
       Psychosomatic Medicine 45 (1983):75-79; Riley, V., "Psychoneuroendocrine influences on
       immunocompetence and neoplasia," *Science* 212 (1981):1100-8.
166   Ornish, Dean, et al., "Can lifestyle changes reverse coronary heart disease?," *The Lancet* 336
       (1990):129-33.
167   Hegsted, M., et al., "Urinary calcium and calcium balance in young men as affected by
       level of protein and phosphorus intake," *Journal of Nutrition* 3 (1981):553-62; Ellis, F.,
       "Incidence of osteoporosis in vegetarians and omnivores," *American Journal of Clinical
       Research* 25 (1972):555; Anand, C., et al., "Effect of protein intake on calcium balance of
       young men given 500 mg calcium daily," *Journal of Nutrition* 104 (1974):695-700.
168   Masess, R., "Bone-mineral content of North American Eskimoes," *American Journal of
       Clinical Nutrition* 27 (1980):916-25.
169   *American Journal of Clinical Nutrition*, (ROH), p 145.

170   Zemel, M., "Calcium utilization: effect of varying level and source of dietary protein,"
       American Journal of Clinical Nutrition 48 (1988):880-83; Breslau, N., "Relationship of animal-
       protein-rich diet to kidney stone formation and calcium metabolism," *Journal of Clinical
       Endocrinology and Metabolism* 66 (1988):140-46.

171   Remer, Thomas, et al., "Estimation of the renal net acid excretion by adults consuming
       diets containing variable amounts of protein," *American Journal of Clinical Nutrition* 59
       (1994):1356-61.

172   *Oakland Tribune* "Every Body Still Needs Milk," August 14, 1997, A:1.

173   Messina, Virginia; Messina, Mark, *The Vegetarian Way* (New York: Crown Trade
       Paperbacks, 1996).

174   *Surgeon General's Report on Nutrition and Health*, U.S. Department of Health and Human
       Services, DHHS (PHS) Publication No. 88-50210:1988.

175   Hernandez-Avila, Mauricio, et al., "Caffeine, moderate alcohol intake, and risk of fractures
       of the hip and forearm in middle-aged women," *American Journal of Clinical Nutrition* 54
       (1991):157-63.

176   Stavric, B., "An update on research with coffee/caffeine," *Food and Chemical Toxicology* 30
       (1992):533-55.

177   Danielson, C., et al., "Hip fractures and fluoridation in Utah's elderly population," *Journal
       of the American Medical Association* 268 (1992):746-47; Sowers, M.F.R., et al., "A prospective
       study of bone mineral content and fracture in communities with different fluoride expo-
       sure," *American Journal of Epidemiology* 134 (1991):649-60.

178   Dalsky, G. "Weight-bearing exercise training and lumbar bone mineral content in post-
       menopausal women," *Annals of Internal Medicine* 108 (1988):824-38.

179   Chow, R., "Effect of two randomized exercise programs on bone mass of healthy post-
       menopausal women," *British Medical Journal* 295 (1987):1441-44.

180   DeMarco, Carolyn, "Take charge of your body" *Women's Health Advisor* (Winlaw, B.C.,
       Canada:Well Women Press, 1994).

181   Heidrich, Ruth, *A Race for Life* (Honolulu: Hawaii Health Publishers,).

182   "Exercise and other factors in the prevention of hip fracture: The Leisure World Study,"
       Epidemiology 1.2 (1991):16.

183   Nilsson, B., "Bone density in athletes," *Clinical Orthopedics* 77 (1971):170-182

184   Lane, N., "Long distance running, bone density, and osteoarthritis," *Journal of the American
       Medical Association* 255 (1986):1147-51.

185   Hitchcox, Lee, *Long Life Now* (Berkeley: Celestial Arts, 1996), p. 84.

186   Ibid, p. 87.

187   Rose, D.P., et al., "International comparisons of mortality rates for cancer of the breast,
       ovary, prostate, and colon, and per capita food consumption," *Cancer* 58 (1986):2363.

188   Rose, D.P., "Dietary fiber and breast cancer," *Nutrition and Cancer*, 13 (1990):1-8; Holm, L.E.,
       et al, "Dietary habits and prognostic factors in breast cancer," *Journal of the National Cancer
       Institute* 81 (1989):1218-23;
       Brisson, J., et al, "Diet, mammographic features of breast tissue, and breast cancer risk"
       American Journal of Epidemiology 130 (1989):14-24.

189   Adlercreutz, H., et al., "Effects of dietary components, including lignans and phytoestro-
       gens, on enterohepatic circulation and liver metabolis, of estrogens and on sex hormone
       binding globulin (SHBG)," *Journal of Steroid Biochemistry* 27 (1987):1135-44.; Kato, T., et al.,
       "Loss of heterocyclic amine mutagens by insoluble hemicellulose fiber and high-molecu-
       lar-weight soluble polyphenolics of coffee," *Mutation Research* 246 (1991):169-78; Rose, D.P.,
       "Dietary prevention of breast cancer," *Medical Oncology and Tumor Pharmacotherapy* 7
       (1990):121-30; Hughes, R.E., "Hypothesis: A new look at dietary fiber," *Human Nutrition:
       Clinical Nutrition* 40 (1986):81-86; Holl, M.H., et al., "Gut bacteria and etiology of cancer of
       the breast," *The Lancet* 2 (1971):172-73.

190   Hankin, Jean H., "Role of nutrition in women's health: Diet and breast cancer," *Journal of the American Dietetic Association* 93 (1993):994-98.

191   Ibid.

192   Fotsis, T., et al., "Genestein, a dietary-derived inhibitor of invitro angiogenesis," *Proceedings of the National Academy of Sciences* 90 (1993):2690-4.

193   "A cautious awe greets drugs that eradicate tumors in mice," *New York Times*, Sunday May 3, 1998, A:1.

194   Bracke, Marc, "The citrus flavanoid tangeretin enhances cell-cell adhesion and inhibits invarions of human MCF-7/6 breast carcinoma cells," paper presented at the 208th American Chemical Society National Meeting, August 21, 1994, Washington, DC.

195   *YES: A Journal of Positive Futures*, Spring 1998, p.11.

196   Sanders, T.A.B., et al., "Hematological studies on vegans," *British Journal of Nutrition* 40 (1978):9-15.

197   Melina, Vesanto, et al., *Becoming Vegetarian* (Summertown: Book Publishing Company, 1995).

198   Gibbs, Gary, *The Food That Would Last Forever* (New York: Avery, 1993).

199   Free radicals are highly unstable molecules that contain an unpaired electron. They are formed when molecules within cells react with oxygen (become oxidized) during normal metabolism, and by way external sources such a radiation and environmental pollution. Without antioxidants to keep them in check, free radical production could ultimately damage cell membranes, DNA, or chromosomes and thereby heighten risk of cancer, heart disease, and aging.

200   Block, G., "Fruit, vegetables and cancer prevention: A review of the epidemiological evidence," *Nutrition and Cancer* 18 (1992):1-29; Block, G., "Vitamin C and cancer prevention: The epidemiologic evidence," *American Journal of Clinical Nutrition* 53 (1991):270S-82S.

201   Ibid.

202   Willet, W.C., et al., "Prediagnostic serum selenium levels and risk of cancer," *The Lancet* 2 (1983):130-34.

203   Meydani, S.N., et al., "Vitamin E supplementation and in vivo immune response in healthy subjects," *Journal of the American Medical Association* 227 (1997):1380-86.

204   Robertson, J., et al., "A possible role for Vitamins C and E in cataract prevention," *American Journal of Clinical Nutrtion* 53 (1991):346S-51S.

205   Borek, C., "Molecular mechanisms in cancer induction and prevention," *Environmental Health Perspectives* 101 (suppl. 3) (1993):237-45.

206   Clark, L., et al., "Effects of selenium supplementation for cancer prevention in patients with carcinoma of the skin," *Journal of the American Medical Association* 276 (1996):1957-63.

207   Borek, C., "Molecular mechanisms in cancer induction and prevention," *Environmental Health Perspectives* 101 (suppl. 3) (1993):237-45.

208   King, Roger A., et al., "Plasma and urinary kinetics of the isoflavones daidzein and genestein after a single soy meal in humans," *American Journal of Clinical Nutrition* 67 (1998):867-72.

209   Ames, Bruce, "Ranking possible carcinogenic hazards," *Science* 236 (1987):272.

210   Elderkin, Susan, et al., *"Forbidden Fruit: Illegal Pesticides in the U.S. Food Supply,"* (Washington, DC: Environmental Working Group, 1995), p. 15.

211   Smith, C., and Beckman, S., *"Export of Pesticides from U.S. Ports in 1990: Focus on Restricted Pesticide Exports"* A Report to the Committee on Agriculture in Science and Education 20 (Sept. 1991).

212   Colborn, Theo, et al., *Our Stolen Future* (New York: Dutton, 1996).

213   Hitchcox, DC, Lee, *Long Life Now* (Berkeley: Celestial Arts, 1997), p. 222.

214   "Is Your Food Safe?" Transcript, CBS News, *48 Hours*, (Burley's Information Services, March 20, 1994), p. 18; Environmental Working Group, "Washed, Peeled—Contaminated," (Washington, D C: EWG, 1994).

215   Mott, Abraham M., "Your Daily Dose of Pesticides Residues" (San Francisco: Pesticide Action Network).

216   Allen, Ruth, et al., "Breast cancer and pesticides in Hawaii: The need for further study," *Environmental Health Perspectives* 105 (Suppl. 3) (1997):679-83.

217   *Rachel's Environment and Health Weekly*, #547, The Weybridge Report, May 22, 1997, Environmental Research Foundation, Annapolis, MD.

218   Center for Science in the Public Interest, *Nutrition Action Healthletter* 24 (June 1997):7.

219   As per note 211.

220   Kaiser, John D., *Immune Power* (New York: St. Martin's Press, 1993), p.27.

221   *Journal of Applied Nutrition* 45 (1993).

222   Center for Science in the Public Interest, *Nutrition Action Health Letter* 24 (1997):4-7.

223   *San Francisco Chronicle*, February 2, 1994, A:6.

224   Steingraber, Sandra, *Living Downstream* (New York: Addison Wesley, 1997).

225   Swanson, Christine, et al., "Alcohol consumption and breast cancer risk among women under age 45 years," *Epidemiology* 8 (1997):231-37; Rosenberg, L., et al., "Breast cancer and alcoholic beverage consumption," *Lancet* 1 (1982):267; Longnecker, Mathew, "Do hormones link alcohol with breast cancer?," 85 (1993):692-93; Ewertz, Marianne, "Alcohol consumption and breast cancer risk in Denmark," *Cancer Causes and Controls* 2 (1991): 247-52; Kato, I., et al., "Alcohol consumption in cancers of hormone related organs in females," *Japan Journal of Clinical Oncology* 19 (1989):202-7.

226   Reichman, Marsha, et al., *Journal of the National Cancer Institute* 85 (1993):722-27.

227   Longnecker, M. P., et al., "A meta-analysis of alcohol consumption in relation to risk of breast cancer," *Journal of the American Medical Association* 260 (1988):652-56.

228   Reichman, M.E., et al., "Effects of alcohol consumption on plasma and urinary hormone concentrations in premenopausal women," *Journal of the National Cancer Institute* 85 (1993):722-7.

229   MacGregor, R. R., "Alcohol and immune defense," *Journal of the American Medical Association* 256 (1986):1474-79.

230   Center for Disease Control "Prevalence of sedentary lifestyle—behavioral risk surveillance system," MMWR 1991, Unites States Government Printing Office.

231   Blair, S., et al., "Physical fitness and all cause mortality: A prospective study of healthy men and women," *Journal of the American Medical Association* 262 (1989):2395-2401.

232   Bernstein, L., et al., "Physical exercise and reduced risk of breast cancer in young women," *Journal of the National Cancer Institute* 86 (1994):1403-08; Frisch, R. E., et al., "Lower prevalence of breast cancer and cancers of the reproductive system among former college athletes compared to non-athletes," *British Journal of Cancer* 52 (1985):885-91. Jacobs, N.M., *Exercise, Calories, Fat and Cancer* (New York: Plenum Press, 1992), Freidenreich, C.M., et al., "Physical activity and risk of breast cancer," *European Journal of Cancer Prevention* 4 (1995):145-51; Simopoulus, A. P., et al., "Energy imbalance and cancer of the breast, colon, and prostate," *Medical Oncology and Tumor Pharmacotherapy*, 7 (1990):109-20. Albanes, D., et al., "Physical activity and risk of cancer in the HANES I population," *American Journal of Public Health*, 79 (1989):744-50; Frisch, R. E., et al., "Lower prevalence of breast cancer and cancers of the reproductive system among former college athletes compared to non-athletes," *British Journal of Cancer*, 52 (1985):885-91.

233   Thune, I., et al., "Physical activity and the risk of breast cancer," *New England Journal of Medicine* 336 (1997):1269-75.

234   Notelovitz, M., and Tonnessen, D., *Menopause and Midlife Health* (New York: St. Martin's, 1993).

235   Colborn, Theo; Dumanoski, Dianne; and Peterson Myers, John, *Our Stolen Future* (New York: Dutton, 1996), p. 218.

236   Raloff, J., "Additional sources of dietary estrogens," *Science News* 6 (1995).

237   American Cancer Society *Cancer Facts and Figures*—1993, p. 14.

238   Colborn, Theo; Dumanoski, Dianne; and Peterson Myers, John, *Our Stolen Future* (New York: Dutton, 1996)

239   Murphy, John, "Risky Business," *The Amicus Journal* 20 Spring (1998):23-27.

240   Herman, Marcia E., "Secondary sexual characteristics and menses in young girls seen in office practice: A study from the Pediatric Research in Office Settings Network," *Pediatrics* 99 (1997):505-12.

241   Hankin, Jean H., "Role of nutrition in women's health: Diet and breast cancer," *Journal of the American Dietetic Association* 93 (1993):994-98.

242   Boyce, Nell, "Growing up too soon," *New Scientist* August 2, (1997):5.

243   Physicians Committee for Responsible Medicine, *Good Medicine* 5 (1996):4.

244   "Overexposed: Organophosphate Insecticides in Children's Food," 1998. Environmental Working Group; Associated Press, January 29, 1998. Contacts: EWG, 1718 Connecticut Ave, N.W., Suite 600, Washington, DC 20009; phone (202) 667-6982; fax (202) 232-2592; email info@ewg.org; website: www.ewg.org; Pesticide Action Network, 49 Powell St., Ste. 500, San Francisco, CA 94102; phone (415) 981-1771; email panna@panna.org; website: http://www.panna.org.

245   *San Francisco Chronicle*, Thursday, Jan. 8, 1998, A:21.

246   Pogoda, Janice M., et al., "Household pesticides and risk of pediatric brain tumors," *Environmental Health Perspectives* 105 (1997):1214-1220.

247   Vom Saal, Frederick S., et al., "A physiologically based approach to the study of bisphenol-A and other estrogenic chemicals on the size of reproductive organs, daily sperm production, and behavior," *Toxicology and Industrial Health* 14 (1998):239-60.

248   Bernstein, L., et al., "The effects of moderate physical activity on menstual cycle patterns in adolescence: Implications for breast cancer prevention," *British Journal of Cancer* 55 (1987):681.

249   Dees C., et al., "Estrogenic-damaging activity of Red No. 3 in human breast cancer cells," *Environmental Health Perspectives* 103 (1997):625-32.

250   Block, Gladys, et al., "Fruits, Vegetables, and Cancer Prevention: A review of the epidemiological evidence," *Nutrition and Cancer* 18 (1992):1-20.

251   Messina, M., et al., "The role of soy products in reducing risk of cancer," *Journal of the National Cancer Institute* 83 (1991):541-46.

252   Messina, M., et al., "Soy intake and cancer risk: A review of the in vitro and in vivo data," *Nutrition and Cancer* 21 (1994):113-31.

253   Lee, H.P., et al., "Dietary effects on breast cancer in Singapore," *The Lancet* 337 (1991):1197-1200.

254   Fotsis, T., et al., "Genestein, a dietary-derived inhibitor of invitro angiogenesis," *Proceedings of the National Academy of Sciences* 90 (1993):2690-94.

255   Schweigerer, L., et al., "Angiogenesis and angiogenesis inhibitors in pediatric disease," *European Journal of Pediatrics* 151 (1992):472-76.

256   Aldercreutz, H., et al., "Dietary phytoestrogens and cancer in vitro and in vivo studies," *Journal of Steroid Biochemistry and Moleculer Biology* 41 (1992):331-37.

257   Kiguchi, K., et al., "Genestein-induced cell differentiation and protein-linked DNA strand breakage in human melanoma cells," *Cancer Communication* 2 (1990):271-77.

258   Yan, L., et al., *Cancer and Nutrition* 29 (1997):1-6.

259   Murkies, A. L., et al., "Dietary flour supplementation decreases postmenopausal hot flashes: Effect of soy and wheat," *Maturitas* 21 (1950):189-95.

Index

ABOUT THE CHEF

Born in France, Jean-Marc Fullsack was trained in classical French cuisine at the Hotel and Restaurant School in Strasbourg. His cooking experience in the United States has included such premiere restaurants as Lutèce in New York, Compound in Santa Fe, L'Ermitage Hotel in Beverly Hills, and the Metropolitan Club in San Francisco.

Jean-Marc was the Chief instructor at the California Culinary Academy in San Francisco, until joining Dr. Dean Ornish's Open Your Heart program at the Preventive Medicine Research Institute. Jean-Marc has prepared dinner at the White House and has personally instructed the chefs about low-fat cooking in the kitchens of the White House, Air Force One, Camp David, and the Navy aircraft carrier, the USS Carl Winson. His recipes and cooking wisdom have been published in numerous magazines, including *Eating Well*, *Sunset*, *Vegetarian Times*, and the books *Eat More, Weigh Less*, and *Every Day Cooking with Dr. Dean Ornish*. Jean-Marc is currently the Executive Chef Instructor at the University of San Francisco Hospitality Management Program and Wellness Center.

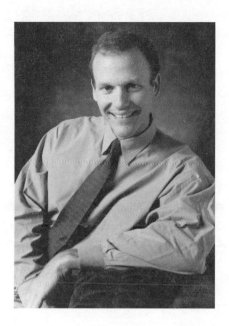

ABOUT THE AUTHOR

Dr. Joseph Keon's commitment to wellness began at the age of 14 when he discovered an abandoned weight set in the family garage. Starting from the time he brought his high school classmates home to share his weights and insight, he has continually refined his natural teaching skills. A wellness consultant for over 18 years, he holds a doctorate degree in nutrition and Fitness Expert certifications by both the Cooper Institute for Aerobics Research and the American Council on Exercise. Dr. Keon is the author of *Whole Health: The Guide to Wellness of Body and Mind* (Parissound, 1997) and co-author of the forthcoming book *Questions That Matter* (Epiphany, 1999). He lives in Mill Valley, California.

ORDER FORM

FAX ORDERS:
(415) 381-5374

TOLL-FREE TELEPHONE ORDERS:
(888) 544-LIFE

MAIL ORDERS:
Parissound Publishing
16 Miller Avenue, Suite 203
Mill Valley, CA 94941 USA

☐ **Whole Health: The Guide to Wellness of Body and Mind ($24.00)**

☐ **The Truth About Breast Cancer: A 7-Step Prevention Plan ($18.00)**

NAME

ADDRESS

CITY   STATE   ZIP CODE

PHONE (   )

PAYMENT (CHECK ONE):

☐ CHECK   ☐ VISA   ☐ MASTERCARD

CARD NUMBER:

NAME ON CARD: EXP. DATE:

SIGNATURE

SHIPPING:

U.S. Priority Mail (2–3 days) $3.00

Bookrate   (2 weeks) $2.30

PRICE:	QUANTITY:	AMOUNT:
$18.00	X	
$24.00	X	
SHIPPING (SEE RATES AT LEFT)		
SUBTOTAL		
SALES TAX (ADD 7.25% IN CA)		
TOTAL		